KT-393-931

energy food

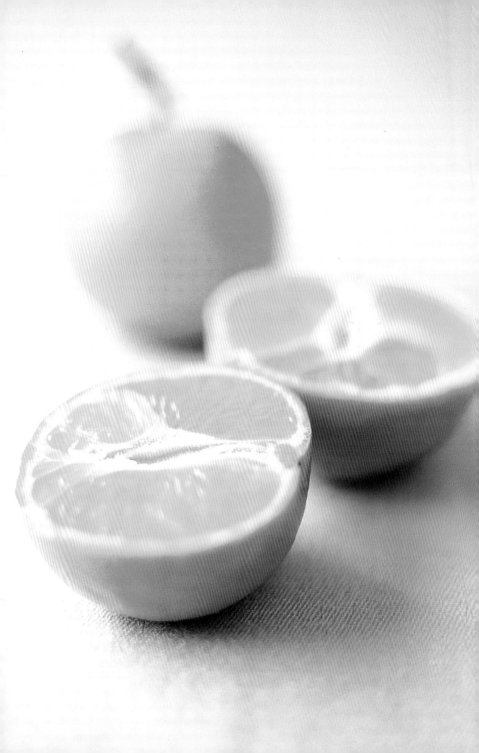

energy food

Sophie Braimbridge
Jenny Copeland SRD

photography by
Deirdre Rooney

MURDOCH
B O O K S

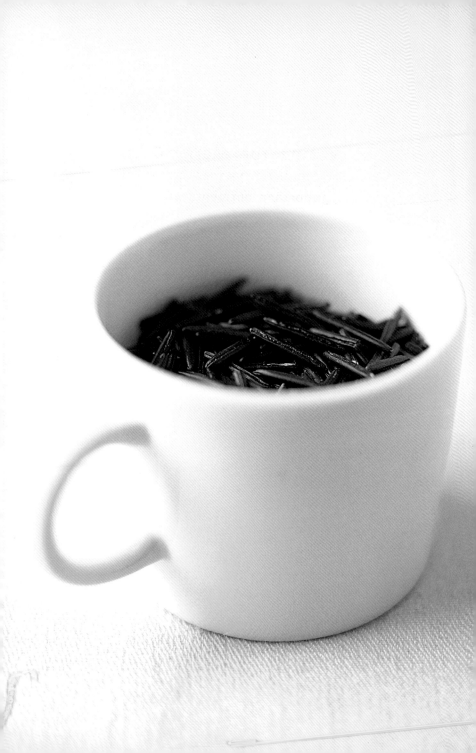

contents

eating for energy

Our current lifestyle, working long hours both in and outside the home and juggling all the demands placed upon us, often pushes our body to its limits. Many people have little time to rest or prepare nutritious meals. Consequently, our energy levels and well-being suffer, making us tired, run down, and vulnerable to infection and poor health. However, making time to care properly for your body with a healthy diet and lifestyle will give you renewed energy and make you feel fantastic.

Every second of our life, thousands of chemical reactions occur in the body, producing enough energy to keep us warm, fuel our brains, allow us to breathe, pump our hearts, and drive all the processes needed to keep us alive. Our body can grow new cells, fight infections, power muscles... yet we take all this for granted – when we are healthy.

This book provides you with information about healthy eating habits and nutritious foods that will give you the energy to get the most out of life. This will help you to cope with a full and busy lifestyle, and enjoy improved vitality and well-being. You will also learn about the effects of specific foods on energy levels and nutritional strategies for alleviating common health problems that cause fatigue and sap your energy.

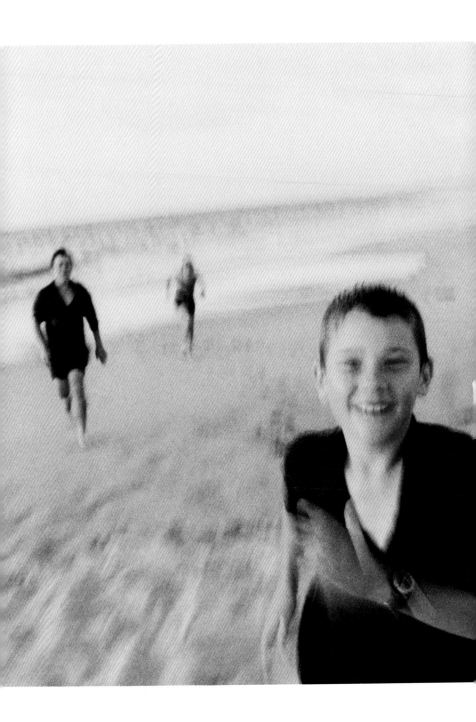

energy from food

Food provides all the energy your body needs. The process is complex, involving a fine balance of energy consumed – measured in calories or joules – and energy produced by your body to power its functions and activities.

FOOD AS FUEL

All foods and most drinks contain calories, which can be used by the body as an energy source. The nutrients that provide us with energy (calories) are carbohydrates, fats and protein (plus alcohol). Different foods and drinks contain different amounts of these nutrients, which are broken down by the body in different ways, and therefore provide different amounts of energy.

The food we eat also provides us with essential vitamins and minerals that we need in order to stay alive, function well, feel energized and stay healthy.

* **Carbohydrates** are the starches and sugars found in plant foods such as fruit, vegetables, pulses and cereals, and are the body's main energy source. All carbohydrates are broken down relatively quickly into simple sugars by digestion and provide the body with a fast fuel source. For optimum health, it is recommended that over half our daily energy requirement (calorie intake) should come from carbohydrates.

Fresh (or dried) fruit and vegetables, dairy products and cereals provide natural sugar for energy as well as vitamins and minerals, and fibre – unlike refined sugar, which provides energy (calories) but no other nutrients. It is therefore better to eat foods that contain natural sugars (fruit) rather than processed, refined ones (such as biscuits and sweets).

* **Fats** are found in animal foods such as meat and dairy products, as well as oils, nuts and seeds, and many processed foods. Fats contain more calories per gram than any other nutrient. Although eating too much fat can lead to health problems, the body uses some energy from fat as a back-up fuel when carbohydrate levels begin to fall.

ENERGY CONTENT OF FOOD

The amount of energy available in food is measured in calories (1 kcal – 1000 calories), or in joules (1 kilojoule/kJ – 1000 joules).

1 kilocalorie = 4.2 kilojoules (approx.)

The amount of energy or kJ in a food is determined by its fat, protein and carbohydrate content. Fat contains twice as many calories as the same amount of carbohydrates or protein.

	kcals/1g	kJ/1g
Carbohydrate	4	16
Fat	9	37
Protein	4	17
Alcohol	7	29

A BALANCED DIET

A balanced diet based on a variety of foods from each major food group will help to keep you feeling healthy and energized. Most of your intake should be carbohydrate-rich foods such as bread, cereals and potatoes rather than fatty or sugary foods. Try to base all your meals and snacks on low-fat, carbohydrate-rich foods and make sure you get some good quality protein each day. Vitamins and minerals also play a role in enhancing vitality, but supplements are generally unnecessary if you eat a balanced diet. In addition, it is much better to get these nutrients from natural food sources (rather than from supplements) as they are absorbed and used more efficiently by the body.

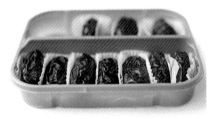

* **Protein** is found in animal foods such as meat, fish, eggs and cheese, as well as in cereals, nuts and pulses. It is needed for cell growth, repair and maintenance. Less readily used as fuel than carbohydrates or fats, protein is utilized by the body when stores of other nutrients fall.

HOW MUCH ENERGY DO YOU NEED?

The amount of energy your body needs depends on your age, activity, gender, health, genetics and metabolic rate (which can be influenced by your physical activity levels and dietary habits). Adults of normal weight usually require around 2000 – 2200 kcals / 8400 – 9240kJ daily. Eating a variety of healthy foods each day should supply you with the optimum ratio of nutrients to meet your energy needs.

THE DAILY DIET

The ideal balance is to eat daily:

* at least 6 servings of starchy carbohydrate foods such as bread, cereals, rice, pasta (all preferably wholegrain) and potatoes.
* at least 5 servings of fruit and vegetables.
* 2–3 servings of dairy products such as milk, or alternatives such as yoghurt, cheese or calcium-enriched soya milk.
* 2 servings of meat, poultry and fish, or alternatives such as eggs, beans, nuts or tofu
* At least 6–8 glasses of water
* 15–25g (½–1oz) of fats and oils (preferably omega-3 enriched – see page 11)

important nutrients

CARBOHYDRATES

Carbohydrates are converted by the body into glucose sugar – the main energy source for the brain and muscles. Any glucose not needed immediately is stored as glycogen in the liver and muscles, and can be released for energy between meals. During exercise, glycogen is broken down into glucose by the muscles to fuel them.

Some carbohydrate-rich foods are digested relatively slowly, resulting in a more gradual, sustained release of glucose energy into the blood (low-glycaemic index/GI foods). Other carbohydrates are digested relatively quickly and produce a large and rapid rise in blood sugar (high-glycaemic index/GI foods). This causes a surge of the hormone insulin resulting in a sharp drop in blood sugar, which can lead to fatigue and hunger in some people.

Low GI foods (such as porridge, lentils, yoghurt, pasta and some fruits) have a GI value of 55 or less. High GI foods (such as white bread, cornflakes, and some snack foods) have a GI value of 70 or more. For sustained energy production, good health and easier weight control most of the carbohydrate-rich foods that you consume should have a low GI rating.

FATS

Although fats are a concentrated source of energy, they are less readily used by the body for fuel than carbohydrates. We all need to eat some healthy fats to provide

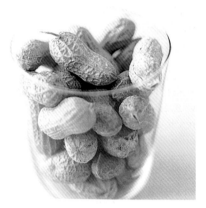

us with fat-soluble vitamins (A, D, E and K) as well as essential fatty acids, which cannot be made in the body (see box, page 11).

The fat in foods is a mixture of three main types:

* **Saturated fats** – found mainly in meat and dairy products as well as in many processed foods. They tend to increase blood cholesterol levels and the risk of heart disease and some cancers.

* **Monounsaturated fats** – found in canola and olive oils, avocados and macadamia nuts.

* **Polyunsaturated fats** – found in oily fish, nuts and seeds and their oils.

Both mono - and polyunsaturated fats can help to reduce blood cholesterol levels if they are eaten in place of saturated fats as part of a low-fat diet.

For good health, it is recommended that fats account for no more than 30% of our total daily energy (calorie) intake – 13% of which should be monounsaturated, 10% polyunsaturated and 7% saturated fat.

PROTEIN

Protein is essential for most of the body's vital functions, including growth, cell repair, and the production of hormones, enzymes and antibodies (the body's messengers and defence agents).

Proteins are made up of chains of amino acids, which contain the essential elements of life – carbon, oxygen, hydrogen and nitrogen (some contain sulphur,

---

ESSENTIAL FATTY ACIDS

* Omega-3 fatty acids are found in oily fish, walnuts and soya, rapeseed (and their oils), as well as green leafy vegetables. They are needed for optimal brain functioning, healthy eyes, can reduce inflammation, and may assist with depression. We require 1–2g per day – equivalent to a 100g (4oz) portion of oily fish, 1–2 teaspoons of vegetable oil or a handful of walnuts.

* Omega-6 fatty acids are found in vegetable oils (particularly olive and sunflower). They keep cells healthy and produce hormones that control functions including growth, blood flow and the immune system. We need around 4g per day (2 teaspoons of sunflower oil or a handful of nuts).

---

too). Tyrosine, an amino acid found in wheatgerm, milk, chocolate, cheese and yoghurt, is used to produce noradrenaline, a hormone that may improve mood.

Protein also triggers the mechanisms that produce the sensation of fullness when we eat. This means that eating some protein with every meal will help to keep hunger at bay between meals.

Animal products like meat, fish, poultry, eggs and dairy products are good sources of protein. Plant foods such as nuts, pulses and cereals (wheat, oats, rice and rye), also contain protein but it may not provide as good a mix of amino acids as protein from animal products. We need around 50g (2oz) of protein per day, which is equivalent to 1 large or 2 small servings of lean meat, chicken, fish or beans.

THE IMPORTANCE OF FLUIDS

In addition to food, your body needs at least 8 large glasses of water every day to function efficiently – even more in hot weather or when exercising. Water is vital for energy production and muscle and brain function. Dehydration causes muscle cramps, tiredness, headaches, and reduces the ability to move, think and react quickly.

Thirst is not a good indication of your fluid needs, because you will already be partially dehydrated before you feel thirsty. To keep your body energized and hydrated it is best to drink small to moderate amounts of fluid regularly during the day.

IMPORTANT VITAMINS AND MINERALS

WHAT IT IS	WHY IT IS NEEDED	WHERE IT IS FOUND
VITAMIN A *(fat soluble)* Preformed vitamin A – in animal foods Provitamin A – in plant foods, can be converted into vitamin A in the body	Interacts with genes to influence cell growth and repair. Helps maintain healthy eyes, skin, hair, nails and mucous membranes, and needed for the immune system. Carotene (plant form of vitamin A) is an important antioxidant that protects against cell damage and possibly some cancers.	Preformed vitamin A: liver, dairy products, eggs, oily fish. Provitamin A: red, orange and yellow fruits; yellow and orange vegetables; dark green leafy vegetables
VITAMIN B1 – thiamin *(water soluble)*	Releases energy from carbohydrates, fats, protein and alcohol. Vital for a healthy nervous system, heart, and normal growth and development. healthy nails, skin and hair. Aids the body's use of other vitamins.	Yeast extract, pork, offal, potatoes, nuts, sunflower seeds, oats, fortified white flour and breakfast cereals
VITAMIN B2 – riboflavin *(water soluble)*	Releases energy from carbohydrates, fats and protein. Vital for normal growth and vision plus immune and nervous systems. Needed for the activity of vitamin B6 and helps to support antioxidants in the body.	Yeast extract, milk, yoghurt, cheese, almonds, eggs, meat, offal, poultry, fish, fortified breakfast cereals
VITAMIN B3 – niacin *(water soluble)*	Needed for release of energy from fats, carbohydrates and protein, mental functioning and healthy skin.	Yeast extract, rice bran, wheat bran, peanuts, liver, oily fish, meat, poultry, rice, barley, fortified cereals
VITAMIN B6 – pyridoxine *(water soluble)*	Needed to release energy from proteins and fats and essential for the healthy function of the nervous and immune systems.	Yeast extract, bananas, avocados, seeds, nuts, legumes, eggs, lean meat, poultry, oily fish
VITAMIN B12 – cyanocobalamin *(water soluble)*	Needed for the formation of DNA and red blood cells, proper growth and for transporting folate into cells.	Meat, liver, poultry, eggs, oily fish, shellfish, dairy products, fortified breakfast cereals

FOLIC ACID (folate) – B group vitamin (water soluble)	Needed for normal cell division, and proper growth and reproduction – essential for the normal development of babies in the womb.	Yeast extract, liver, fortified breakfast cereals, green leafy vegetables, asparagus, pulses, seeds, wheatgerm, wheat bran, oat bran
VITAMIN C – ascorbic acid (water soluble)	Antioxidant which helps prevent cell damage caused by free radicals and pollutants such as cigarette smoke. Essential for healthy skin, bones and teeth. Improves iron absorption and is needed to produce neurotransmitters such as noradrenaline and serotonin and thyroid hormones.	Many fruits (especially citrus, berries, mangoes, kiwi, figs, nectarines) and vegetables (especially peppers, spinach, broccoli, watercress, cauliflower, cabbage, peas, tomatoes, chillies)
VITAMIN E – tocopherols (fat soluble)	Powerful antioxidant that protects the body's cells from damage by free radicals. Required for healing, and healthy nerves and red blood cells.	Oily fish, liver, eggs, dairy produce, vegetable oils, nuts, seeds, peanut butter, wholegrain bread
IRON (mineral)	Essential for healthy red blood cells, oxygen transport, energy production and mental functioning. Also assists with immune functioning	Liver, meat, sardines, eggs, dark green leafy vegetables, fortified breakfast cereals
CHROMIUM (mineral)	Needed for release of energy from fats and carbohydrates, and normal control of blood sugar levels.	Egg yolks, meat, liver, dairy products, nuts, wholegrains, oysters, potatoes, spinach
PHOSPHORUS (mineral)	Maintains bone structure (with calcium and magnesium). Required for almost all metabolic reactions in the body and for energy production.	Yeast extract, meat, liver, poultry, fish, milk, cheese, oysters, nuts, seeds wheat bran, oily fish
MAGNESIUM (mineral)	Needed for the activity of vitamin D and many hormones, for maintaining bone strength, nerve and muscle functioning, and for releasing energy from carbohydrates, fats and protein.	Green leafy vegetables, tofu, seeds, nuts, bananas, wholegrains, wheatgerm, wheat bran

energy for life

Keeping your energy levels high involves eating regular meals that contain the right balance of nutrients and healthy foods, as well as keeping active, spending time outdoors, and getting enough good quality rest.

WHEN TO EAT

Food not only provides the necessary energy and nutrients to keep your body healthy and active, but it can also affect your mood and mental function. As food is broken down in the body, nutrients enter the bloodstream and are transported to the brain and other organs – providing a fresh supply of energy. Eating the right foods at the right time of day can therefore make a difference to your feelings of energy and alertness and can affect your sleeping and relaxation patterns. By adjusting the amount and type of food you eat, as well as the timing of your meals, you can help sustain optimum mental and physical energy when you most need it. For example:

* A low-fat, nutrient-dense breakfast will give rise to a higher level of alertness in the morning, coupled with less physical fatigue and a better mood.
* Some people experience fatigue or a dip in energy after lunch, which may be caused by the food content of the meal. High-protein and high-carbohydrate lunches appear to produce greater alertness and more focused attention; whereas lunches that are high in

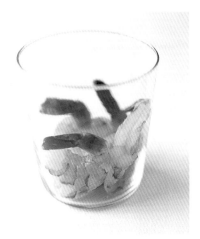

sugar and in fat tend to lead to greater fatigue, sleepiness and distraction.

It is best to tailor your eating patterns to suit your daily activities. You may prefer to 'graze' throughout the day, eating four to six smaller snack-like meals, or to eat only three balanced meals at regular intervals. You can enhance your health and well-being by making sure you drink plenty of

---

ENERGY-BOOSTING SNACKS

* Fish or vegetable sushi box.
* Sardines or tuna on top of wholemeal bread or toast.
* Ryebread spread with low-fat cream cheese or cottage cheese, garnished with watercress or spinach.
* Vegetable extract spread on a toasted crumpet

---

water, undertake regular physical activity and eat healthy, nourishing foods most of the time.

Start by making a series of small changes one at a time over a long period, rather than trying to change all your habits at once. Try cooking a few healthy meals from this book every week. That way, you'll quickly discover how easy it is to cook healthily and how great eating in this way makes you feel.

AVOIDING FATIGUE

* Low blood sugar, low iron levels and dehydration can cause fatigue. Consume energy-boosting snacks and rehydrating fluids to alleviate symptoms.

* Drink plenty of water throughout the day.

* Eat quick snacks such as bananas, dates, raisins and other dried fruits, such as dried apricots, to boost blood sugar levels and stimulate energy production.

* Eat slow-releasing starchy foods such as pasta, brown rice, potatoes and wholemeal bread for a sustained flow of energy – these are a good lunch option.

* Eat fruit and vegetables to provide the vital nutrients for your body to convert into energy, including B vitamins and folate.

* Eat iron- and zinc-rich foods such as lean meat and fish to prevent anaemia and boost your metabolism.

* Cut down on sugary foods, alcohol and caffeinated drinks.

EXERCISE

Sustained exercise such as walking, cycling, swimming, dancing or jogging speeds up your breathing, raises your heart and metabolic rates, and can help burn up body fat. During exercise, blood flow to the brain and muscles increases and adrenalin is released, making you feel more alert and alive. Exercise can also trigger the release of endorphins – chemicals produced by the brain which make you feel happier, calmer and more relaxed. Numerous research studies have shown that regardless of your present level of fitness, regular exercise will help to boost your energy levels and sense of well-being.

During exercise the muscles are fuelled by glucose and fats in the blood, and by glycogen stored in the liver and muscles. In a well-fed person, the muscles normally contain enough glycogen to fuel about 90 –120 minutes of physical activity. These stores can be boosted in preparation for prolonged periods of intense activity such as sports matches, running, rambling or cycling by eating a carbohydrate-rich diet for at least three days prior to the event. This strategy is known as carbohydrate loading and can improve performance and stamina in events of long duration, as it provides extra fuel for the body. In order to make this strategy effective, you should also try to drink plenty of water to aid the processing of nutrients.

STIMULANTS/DEPRESSANTS

* **Caffeine** is a stimulant found in tea, coffee, cocoa and cola drinks that is known to have a powerful affect on alertness and mood. While one cup can initially improve alertness by stimulating an increase in blood sugars and adrenalin, this is only a temporary effect. It is easy to overdose, risking fatigue, anxiety, insomnia and even shaking. Your body can also become used to regular caffeine consumption, so that caffeine becomes less effective with time.

Moderate caffeine consumption (2–3 cups of coffee per day) does not appear to cause problems in most healthy people. If you need to cut down, it is best to do so gradually in order to avoid withdrawal symptoms, such as irritability, nausea, headaches and mood swings. Try spacing out your caffeine drinks over longer and longer intervals, then make them weaker (you can

---

HIGH-CARBOHYDRATE MEALS & SNACKS

* Low-fat pasta, rice, potato or couscous dishes
* Bread, rolls, pitta bread, English muffins, crumpets, fruit bread, bagels – all with little or no butter, margarine or mayonnaise and topped with lean meat, low-fat cheese and salad, jam or honey.
* Bread roll and low-fat soup.
* Low-fat popcorn.
* Low-fat milk or yoghurt.
* Fruit – fresh, dried or tinned (in juice).
* Breakfast cereals, porridge.

LOSING WEIGHT

* If you are trying to lose weight, beware of crash dieting, as this will prevent the body from taking in sufficient calories to maintain its normal functions and energy production, and will usually leave you feeling tired, irritable and hungry. It is better to lose weight slowly – no more than 0.5–1kg (1–2lb) a week – by cutting down your fat intake and eating healthier meals to achieve optimum body weight. Replace high-fat foods with low-fat, carbohydrate-rich foods such as fruit, vegetables, bread, pasta and cereals in sensible amounts.

---

dilute cola with low-calorie lemonade, for example, or with sparkling mineral water) or replace them with fruit juices, mineral water, water, herb teas and non-alcoholic fruit cocktails.

* **Alcohol** can reduce mental performance and disrupt the quality of your sleep, and because it is a toxin it can interfere with your liver and kidney functions. It also robs you of vital nutrients (especially the B vitamins), raises blood pressure, and its diuretic action can dehydrate the body, causing headaches and fatigue. Alcohol is a depressant, and because it contains empty calories – that is, energy without any nutritional value – it can cause weight gain.

* **Smoking** compromises your well-being, robs you of precious energy and can cause serious health problems. Nicotine initially stimulates the brain, then acts as a

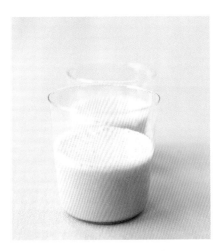

especially in place of healthy meals, can make the problem worse (see page 16).

SLEEP
A lack of good-quality sleep can make you fatigued and irritable, adversely affecting your mood and your ability to deal with stress and work demands. Age and activity levels determine the amount of sleep you need – in general, people tend to need less sleep as they get older. However, it is the quality rather than the quantity of sleep that makes you feel refreshed. Diet and the timing of food consumption can affect the quality of sleep and your ability relax because of the way they affect

depressant. It also increases the rate at which you use B vitamins and vitamin C – smokers may require twice as much vitamin C per day as non-smokers to help counteract the increased numbers of toxins entering the body.

ANXIETY AND STRESS
The impact of anxiety and stress on energy levels should not be underestimated. Excessive amounts of stress over prolonged periods can cause fatigue, digestive problems, lowered immunity, loss of appetite and disturbed sleeping patterns. This can result in weight fluctuations (gain or loss), food cravings, sleep problems and nutrient deficiencies, all of which sap the body's energy levels and rob you of vitality.

Consuming alcohol or excessive amounts of caffeine in coffee, tea and colas,

FOODS TO COMBAT ANXIETY AND STRESS
* Eat balanced, filling meals based on high carbohydrate foods with some lean protein to satisfy your hunger and allow you to deal better with stressful situations.

Foods that may help you manage anxiety and feelings of stress include:

* Meat, eggs, cheese, nuts, wholegrain bread, brown rice and muesli, which are good sources of the B vitamins.

* Fresh fruit and vegetables, which provide vitamin C and other antioxidants and healthy compounds.

* Slightly sweetened milky drinks, such as hot milk and honey, as they contain the protein tryptophan, which may stimulate the production of serotonin, a natural tranquilizer.

digestion and the hormones that regulate other body processes.

Some of our bodily processes operate according to a 24-hour biological clock – a circadian rhythm – meaning that certain functions occur at certain times. Melatonin, a hormone secreted by the pineal gland in the brain, is involved in regulating the body's cycles of sleep and wakefulness, and may also enhance immune function. Serotonin, the 'happy hormone', is needed for the production of melatonin, and also affects mood and the nervous system. Some foods are known to suppress or stimulate the production of these body-controlling hormones. Vitamin B6, for example, aids the production of serotonin, so foods rich in this vitamin (pulses, seeds and bananas) may promote calmness and sleep.

Melatonin levels rise gradually during the evening and then fall again as sunlight levels increase in the morning. Stress can sometimes interfere with this natural process, severely affecting our capacity to sleep and energy levels during the day.

When stressed, our body automatically produces adrenalin – the hormone that raises heartbeat, slows digestion and increases blood sugar levels by releasing glycogen from the liver and muscles. This makes us ready for activity and prevents sleep. Cortisol is another hormone released in times of stress and prolonged activity, which also prevents relaxation. Foods that provide a slow release of energy – low

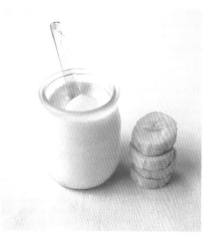

glycaemic index (GI) carbohydrates such as starchy vegetables and wholegrains – will stabilize blood sugar levels, which may be helpful during stressful times (as this prevents large falls in blood sugar). Stimulants such as caffeine, however, can compound stress by increasing the release of adrenalin.

Not eating enough food to satisfy your hunger during the night can result in disrupted sleep. A low-fat evening meal based on low-GI carbohydrates will prevent hunger and keep blood sugar levels stable. Avoid alcoholic and caffeinated drinks in the evening to give you a more restful sleep.

Depression may also disrupt sleep by altering serotonin levels. Low-fat snacks like milky drinks, bananas and yoghurt for supper may alleviate this problem. Food allergies and intolerances that cause digestive problems can also disturb sleep.

energy-depleting conditions

Apart from life's everyday stresses and demands, excessive tiredness and low energy levels can be caused by a number of conditions including food intolerances.

IRON DEFICIENCY

Iron deficiency is a common nutritional problem in Western societies, despite the abundant food supply. It can eventually lead to the more serious condition of anaemia, where the body's iron stores are totally depleted. As iron levels drop, haemoglobin production falls, which means that oxygen transport to the body's tissues is impaired. Symptoms include tiredness, lethargy, dizziness, breathlessness and depression. There may also be a reduction in physical and mental performance, the ability to recover after exercise, cold tolerance, and immune function. Athletes, females, dieters and the elderly also have an increased risk of iron deficiency.

The iron found in animal foods such as meat, liver and fish is absorbed much more efficiently by the body than the iron found in plant foods, such as leafy green vegetables and grains (although the vitamin C found in citrus juice, fruit and vegetables can improve iron absorption from plant sources, as can eating the two types of iron together).

Tannins in tea and coffee can inhibit the absorption of iron, so avoid consuming these drinks with meals. Phytic acid present in pulses, and brans can also inhibit iron absorption, so if you are iron-dficient avoid consuming lots of bran or bran-based cereals. Choose drinking powders and breakfast cereals that are fortified with iron (check the labels) to help boost your iron intake.

Vitamin B12 and folate are also needed for the formation of red blood cells. Folate is found in wholegrain cereals, dark green leafy vegetables, nuts and liver. Vitamin B12 is found in meat, fish, eggs and dairy products, so vegetarians – and especially vegans – may be at risk of a deficiency. If you suspect that you are suffering from an iron or vitamin B12 deficiency, see your doctor for confirmation. Do not self-diagnose or start taking supplements, as this can lead to other health problems.

THE IMMUNE SYSTEM

* A poor diet, a lack of exercise or sleep, pollution and stress can all depress our immune system. Regular exercise boosts circulation, helping oxygen and nutrients travel to the cells to provide greater resistance to viruses and infections. However, many foods and nutrients can help boost the immune system (see chart, pages 12–13), helping to prevent illnesses which sap energy and vitality. The best approach to keeping your immune system functioning well is to eat a healthy, well-balanced diet that will ensure you consume enough of all the important nutrients (see page 9).

POST-VIRAL FATIGUE – MYALGIC ENCEPHALOMYELITIS (ME)

While the causes of ME are still unknown it can occur after a viral infection and results in a decline in energy levels. Symptoms include fatigue, pain, exhaustion, depression, digestive complaints, sleep disturbances, poor concentration and memory loss. The main treatment is rest, certain medications, and eating a healthy, well-balanced diet that contains enough good-quality protein, carbohydrates, vitamins and minerals to assist the body's healing processes. Eating small, regularly spaced meals through-out the day may help improve nutrient absorption and raise energy levels.

Foods such as pasta, wholegrain bread, oats and pulses provide a steady release of energy and can help to reduce fatigue. They also contain fibre to help with digestive problems and B vitamins for a healthy nervous system and energy production. Meat, fish, poultry, eggs and dairy products are good sources of protein and essential for healthy tissues and vitality. Fresh fruits and vegetables provide vitamin C and other antioxidants, which are important during times of stress and illness.

Caffeine may exacerbate the symptoms of ME because it stimulates the nervous system. Alcohol can also worsen symptoms, especially fatigue, and can also deplete the body's supplies of B-group vitamins and vitamin C.

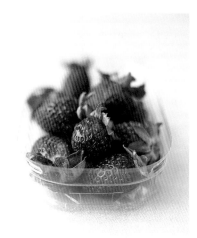

DEPRESSION

Many people suffer from depression at some stage during their life. It not only affects mental well-being and self-esteem, but can seriously reduce energy levels. In most cases, medical intervention, counselling and lifestyle changes are needed to treat depression, but a healthy diet is also very important, since mood can be affected by what you eat. Basing your diet on fresh fruits and vegetables, low-fat cereal and dairy products, lean meats, pulses, eggs, nuts and seeds will ensure you get all nutrients needed to maintain health and a sense of well-being.

Some nutrient deficiencies – including iron, selenium, vitamin B6 and omega-3 fatty acids – are associated with feelings of depression. Consulting a doctor or dietitian can help to determine whether you are suffering from a deficiency. Vitamin B supplements (particularly B6 and B2) have helped alleviate depression in some women taking oral contraceptive pills or suffering from premenstrual syndrome. However, rather than relying on supplements, try to improve your diet first. Simply replacing high-calorie 'junk' foods with healthier foods will help to boost your intake of B vitamins and other beneficial compounds.

Avoiding alcohol (a brain depressant) and excessive caffeine is also important for alleviating depression. Similarly, fatty foods can depress blood sugar levels, mood and alertness, and should therefore be limited.

Depression can lead to a loss of appetite increasing the risk of nutrient deficiencies, which may in turn aggravate the condition – a common problem among the elderly.

Exercise increases the circulation of vital nutrients to the brain. Keeping active with regular exercise and outdoors activities, as well as getting good-quality rest, will recharge your batteries and lift your mood. Even brisk walking for 30 minutes or more at least three times a week helps to produce mood-enhancing chemicals (endorphins).

FOOD INTOLERANCES AND ALLERGIES

Although true food allergies are relatively rare, adverse reactions – food intolerance or sensitivity – to food are fairly common. Some people can experience excessive tiredness due to a food intolerance; other symptoms include digestive upset, skin

SEASONAL AFFECTIVE DISORDER (SAD)

* Some people feel particularly depressed and lethargic during the long, dark winter months. It is thought that this is caused by reduced exposure to sunlight which results in an imbalance of brain neurotransmitters such as serotonin and dopamine (which control mood). As we tend to be less active in winter, we may also be producing fewer endorphins – the body's 'feel good' chemicals. Endorphins are released during exercise and act as natural painkillers, providing a sense of happiness and well-being.

* If you suffer from SAD, ensure you get some natural light by getting out of doors every day.

* Try increasing your physical activity levels to stimulate endorphin production.

* A low-fat, high-carbohydrate diet, with plenty of fresh fruit and vegetables, has also been shown to help. Try eating colourful meals – such as a salad, stew or stirfry made up of red, green and orange peppers (capsicums), tomatoes, courgettes (zucchini), aubergine (eggplant) and sweetcorn, or fruit salads using melons, kiwis, oranges, strawberries and other berries.

* Avoid bingeing on sweets and other sugary foods and eating large servings of protein-rich foods such as meat, poultry, fish and eggs. People suffering from SAD often gain weight during the winter months, so following a low-fat, high-carbohydrate diet, drinking plenty of water and taking exercise is a good way to prevent this.

problems, asthma, hives, eczema, rashes, nausea, headaches, abdominal cramps, flatulence, and constipation or diarrhoea. Food intolerances can occur at any age and susceptibility often changes as we get older. They may be exacerbated by stress, anxiety, medication such as antibiotics, a depressed immune system, or excessive consumption of highly processed foods, artificial colours and additives. Some common food culprits include cow's milk, chocolate, yeast, fish, nuts, wheat, gluten, some fruits and vegetables, and alcohol. Foods that are unlikely to cause intolerance symptoms are pears, lamb, lettuce, apples, rice and carrots.

If you think you have a food intolerance consult your doctor, who may then refer you to a qualified allergy specialist and dietitian. Beware of allergy tests not performed by medical professionals, as many are unproven and can lead to restrictive diets and the use of expensive supplements.

PREMENSTRUAL SYNDROME (PMS)

PMS is characterized by a number of emotional and physiological symptoms that vary greatly between women in both nature and severity. These include fatigue, depression, anxiety, irritability, headaches, changes in sleep and eating patterns, bloating and a drop in energy levels.

In healthy women, a high-carbohydrate diet that is low in fat and protein may help to reduce PMS symptoms, while cutting down on salt intake can help to reduce fluid retention. Ensuring an intake of omega-3 essential fatty acids (found in oily fish and walnuts, for example) has been shown to help reduce menstrual pain.

Chocolate is frequently craved during the premenstrual period and is thought to stimulate the release of some mood-enhancing chemicals. However, it is high in fat and so large amounts are best avoided. Instead, try low-fat options such as low-fat chocolate pudding or yoghurt, or low-fat drinking chocolate, to satisfy your cravings.

Avoid excessive intake of alcohol (depressant) and caffeinated drinks (stimulants) such as tea, coffee, cocoa and colas – as these can exaggerate mood swings and fluid changes in the body.

THYROID DISORDERS

The thyroid gland produces the hormones that control your metabolic rate, growth and development. An underactive thyroid gland causes the body's metabolic rate to slow down, leading to tiredness,

---

USEFUL FOODS FOR THYROID PROBLEMS

* Selenium-rich foods – brazil nuts, kidneys, liver, mussels, clams, scallops, oysters, squid, lobster, prawns, fish from the sea, sunflower seeds, grainy bread, eggs, beef, pork, chicken, wheatgerm and bran.
* Iodine-rich foods – seafood and fish from the sea, seaweed, iodized salt, bread, dairy products, eggs, meat, fruit and vegetables.

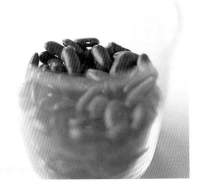

depression, weight gain, sensitivity to cold, constipation and dry skin and hair. Iodine and selenium are essential for the synthesis of thyroid hormones and are found in vitamin B-rich foods such as fish, wholegrains, pulses and seeds.

Chemicals naturally present in raw cabbage, turnips, swedes and cassava can interfere with the body's ability to use iodine for the production of thyroid hormones. However, most of these chemicals are destroyed by cooking and these foods are generally not eaten in large amounts by people in Western societies.

DIABETES

Diabetes is characterized by high blood sugar levels, caused by the body's inability to make sufficient insulin (Type 1 diabetes) and/or the inability of the body's tissues to utilize/recognize insulin (Type 2 diabetes). Insulin is a hormone produced by the pancreas, which is secreted in response to rising blood sugar levels following food consumption and stimulates cells to take up glucose from the blood. Type 1 diabetes is usually diagnosed in childhood; Type 2 diabetes is more common and usually occurs in people over the age of 30 – the risk is increased in those who are overweight, inactive, or have a family history of the condition. Symptoms include tiredness, lethargy, thirst, recurrent infections and, if undiagnosed, eventually serious health problems and death.

Type 2 diabetes can go undiagnosed, as people attribute their symptoms to 'getting old'. However, it can be controlled by diet and exercise alone, or by diet, exercise and medication. A urine and blood test will confirm diabetes, and dietary advice and/or medication tailored to your specific needs by your medical practitioner or dietitian can control the condition. It is especially important to control the amount and type of carbohydrate consumed, as a means of controlling blood sugar levels. High GI carbohydrates and sugary foods and drinks should be avoided, as these quickly raise blood sugar levels. Fat intake, particularly of saturated fats, should also be limited as diabetes significantly increases the risk of heart disease. If you have diabetes, altering your diet to control the condition will give you more energy.

dairy products, alternatives and oils

Dairy products provide us with most of the nutrients needed for energy production, while oils can be good sources of essential fatty acids and fat-soluble vitamins.

* **Milk** is a good source of quality protein, rich in calcium, and contains B vitamins, phosphorus and zinc, which are important for energy production, the immune system and sleep. Skimmed milk contains half the calories of whole milk but retains nearly all its nutritional content. Goat's milk is nutritionally similar to cow's milk, so is a useful substitute for people on a cow's milk-free diet. Milk is used to make a wide range of dairy products, including fromage frais (similar to yoghurt but without the acidic taste). Low-fat versions can be used in recipes for dips, toppings and desserts. Quark is very low in fat and can be used instead of fromage frais. Buttermilk is also low fat with added bacterial cultures to thicken it. It can be used for baking and as a topping for breakfast cereals.

* **Cheese** is a good source of protein and an excellent provider of easily absorbed calcium. It is also an important source of vitamin B12 for vegetarians. Most types are high in fat, however, so should be eaten in moderation. Hard cheeses such as stilton, cheddar and parmesan contain 35% fat; soft cheeses such as camembert and brie around 26%; ricotta only 11% and cottage cheese less than 4% fat. Lower fat varieties are now widely available and the stronger the flavour the less you will need to use for cooking.

* **Soya milk** and rice milk are good alternatives to milk for people who cannot tolerate dairy products or want to avoid eating animal products. Look for brands with added calcium and vitamins B12 and D to ensure you get enough of these nutrients.

* **Vegetable oils** from nuts, seeds and pulses supply essential fatty acids – monounsaturated and polyunsaturated fats, some of which cannot be made by the body. They also increase the body's absorption of fat-soluble vitamins A, D, E and K from other foods. They are high in energy, providing over 100 calories per tablespoon. For good health, use olive, canola, rape- or linseed oils as your major oils, as they provide monounsaturated fat and essential omega-3 fats.

FOCUS ON YOGHURT

* Yoghurt produces a slow, sustained release of glucose energy and is a good source of protein and calcium, especially for people who can't tolerate the lactose in cow's milk as the bacterial cultures used to ferment milk into yoghurt use up the lactose as their energy source.

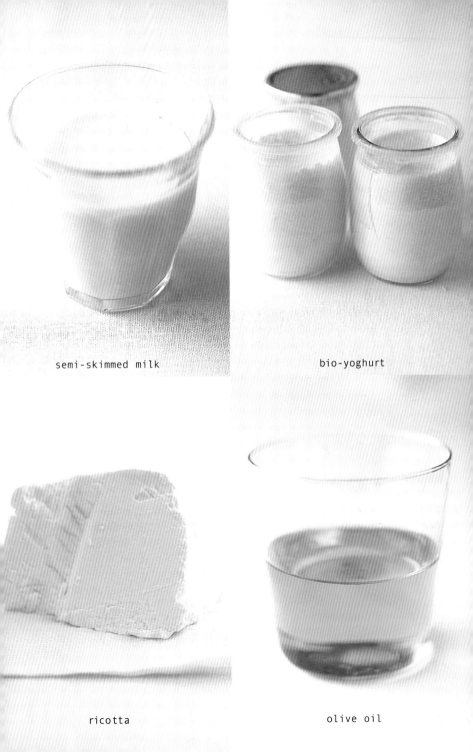

semi-skimmed milk

bio-yoghurt

ricotta

olive oil

meat, poultry, fish and eggs

These foods are excellent sources of protein needed for bodily functions. They also provide vitamins and minerals essential for energy production, such as iron and zinc.

* **Red meat** is a rich source of protein, iron and zinc, the latter two being particularly well absorbed from this source. It also supplies chromium, which is needed for insulin to function properly in the control of blood sugar levels.

* **Liver and kidneys** are highly nutritious foods and the richest source of iron and vitamin B12, needed for healthy blood production and the prevention of anaemia, which increases fatigue and susceptibility to illness. Small to moderate portions every now and again can give you a good nutrient boost.

* **Poultry** is low in fat (if the skin is avoided), and provides minerals and some B vitamins. Both chicken and fish are excellent sources of protein to help sustain energy levels.

* **Oily fish** include sardines, mackerel, tuna and salmon. They contain high levels of essential omega-3 fats.

* **Tuna**, whether fresh or tinned, provides good-quality protein, a good range of minerals and B vitamins, and omega-3 essential fatty acids.

* **Sardines** are a good source of protein and calcium (if eaten with the bones), a range of other minerals and vitamins, and omega-3 fatty acids if tinned in water or sauce (not oil).

* **Salmon** is a good source of omega-3 essential fatty acids and many minerals, including calcium if eaten with the bones.

* **Non-oily fish** such as cod, sea bass and haddock are lower in fat and calories than oily fish but are still excellent sources of protein and other essential nutrients.

* **Eggs** provide iron, zinc, calcium, B vitamins and protein, so are excellent for energy production. Contrary to popular belief, they are relatively low in fat (if not fried). Although a source of dietary cholesterol, this is not well absorbed by the body and does not cause blood cholesterol levels to rise significantly. Up to one egg per day is fine unless you have a high blood cholesterol level.

FOCUS ON PROTEIN

*Although we can obtain protein from vegetarian sources such as beans, pulses, grains and nuts, these plant foods (with the exception of soya) don't contain all the amino acids needed by the body. Animal sources contain more protein per gram and all the essential amino acids in the proportions required. However, eating too much animal protein can cause weight gain as the excess is transformed into fat. Adults usually need only 1–2 servings of protein-rich foods daily.

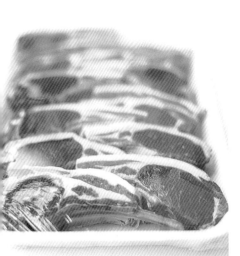

lamb

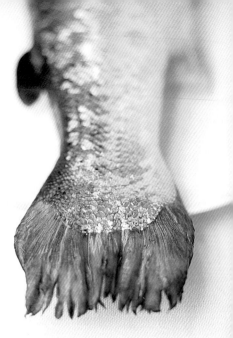

salmon

eggs

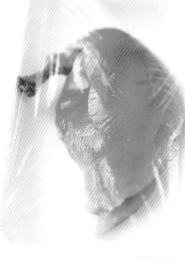

chicken

pulses or legumes

One of the most versatile and nutritious food groups, pulses or legumes are good sources of protein, carbohydrate, fibre, B-group vitamins and many minerals.

Beans and pulses are especially good sources of soluble fibre – which slows down the absorption of glucose into the bloodstream preventing a sudden rise in blood sugar levels. This gradual release of fuel is good for sustaining energy levels and the sense of fullness. Soluble fibre acts by retaining water in the gut like a sponge, speeding up the passage of waste products and increasing the gut's motility. This prevents bowel problems such as constipation, which can effect energy levels and wellbeing. Whole, mashed or puréed beans and pulses add flavour and texture as well as important nutrients to many different dishes, and are a nutritious alternative to meat. They are low in fat and contain no cholesterol.

* **Lentils**, both green and brown, are excellent sources of fibre, minerals and slow-release carbohydrate for sustained energy. They are very filling and make delicious soups, curries and bakes.

* **Soya beans** are a good source of protein, fibre, B vitamins including folate, and the minerals potassium, phosphorus, iron and calcium. Products containing them, such as tofu and tempeh, are useful in a wide range of recipes. Miso and soy sauce make good flavourings.

* **Bean sprouts** are actively growing seedlings and therefore retain more of their nutrients than other vegetables, which start to lose their vitamin content as soon as they are picked. Most commonly sprouted are mung beans, but lentils, aduki beans, chickpeas and soya beans are all used for sprouting. Cook soya sprouts before eating to destroy toxins and chickpea sprouts to make them tender. A big bowl of mixed bean sprouts with an accompanying low-fat sauce is a delicious and nutritious light meal. Alternatively add them to salads, stir-fries or sandwiches.

FOCUS ON VEGETARIAN DIETS

* Some of the essential minerals and vitamins we need are most readily available from meat and fish, so it is vital that vegetarians consume a good amount of non-meat foods that are rich in iron, vitamin B12 and folate in order to avoid fatigue and iron deficiency or even anaemia. Non-meat sources of these nutrients include beans and pulses, wholegrain cereals, nuts, eggs, dried fruits and dark green leafy vegetables for iron; dairy products for vitamin B12; and fruit, vegetables, nuts and grains for folate.

yellow split peas

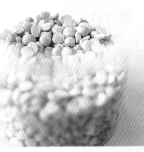

red kidney beans

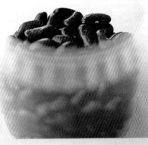

chickpeas

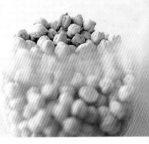

lentils

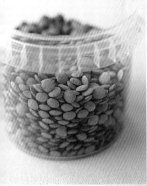

tofu

soya beans

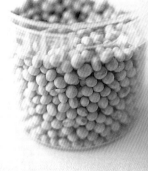

flageolet beans

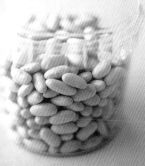

tempeh

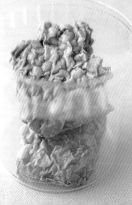

butter beans

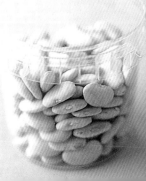

nuts and seeds

Nuts and seeds are good sources of protein, fibre, vitamin E, B vitamins, many minerals including phosphorus, iron, copper and potassium – and energy (calories) from fat.

* **Nuts** and nut oils are high in calories which makes them a concentrated source of energy. Most of their calories come from fat – usually around 50% – but this is mainly unsaturated fat (poly- or mono-unsaturated fats) which provides essential fatty acids – omega-3 and omega-6 – needed by the body for optimum health. A handful of nuts daily will provide all of the body's omega-6 needs. Nuts are also high in protein and are one of the richest vegetable sources of vitamin E. However, roasting nuts, while enhancing their flavour, may destroy their vitamin E and thiamin content. Avoid salted and oil-roasted varieties – choose dry-roasted or raw nuts instead. Walnut, hazelnut, sesame, almond and macadamia nut oils are now available.

* **Almonds** provide many minerals including calcium if eaten with their skin on. Try them whole, flaked, blanched, chopped or ground.

* **Brazil nuts** are the richest food source of selenium – a powerful antioxidant.

* **Walnuts** are the only nuts rich in omega-3 essential fatty acids which are needed for optimal brain functioning.

* **Seeds**, like nuts, are nutrient and energy dense as they are high in protein, fibre, vitamins, minerals and unsaturated fats. They contain around 100 calories per tablespoon.

* **Pumpkin seeds** are rich in minerals needed for energy-producing processes. They are delicious toasted and added to bread, fruit salads and yoghurts. Snacking on small amounts will give you an energy and nutrient boost.

* **Sesame seeds** are rich in phosphorus, calcium and vitamin E, making them a useful addition to dairy-free diets. They can be used to make tahini – the dark version has the strongest flavour and the most calcium – which can be blended with chickpeas to make hummus, a delicious energy-boosting snack with vegetables or on toast.

* **Sunflower seeds** are useful sources of vitamin E and zinc.

FOCUS ON ALLERGIES

* Nuts – especially peanuts – are potential food allergens. Although relatively rare, peanut allergy usually arises in infancy and can last for life. Sufferers should avoid all foods containing traces of nuts – including nut oils and blended oils, and foods manufactured in factories that use nuts as raw ingredients, as there is a danger of cross-contamination.

peanuts

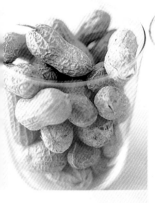

pumpkin seeds

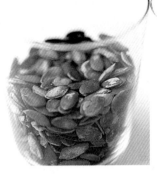

almonds

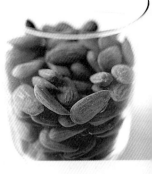

sunflower seeds

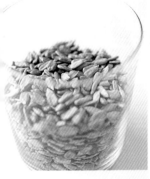

sesame seeds

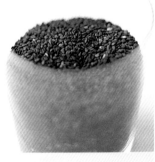

linseeds

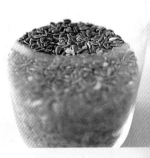

brazil nuts

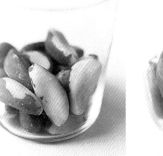

chestnuts

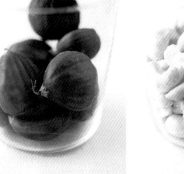

cashew nuts

breads, cereals and grains

Grains and grain products are a major source of starchy carbohydrate for energy, fibre for bulk and bowel function, and B vitamins for energy and a healthy nervous system.

Cereals and grains are low in fat, free from cholesterol, and contain a range of minerals and other healthy plant compounds, including antioxidants. They are an excellent source of complex, starchy carbohydrate, vital for energy production, and are used in foods such as bread, pasta and cakes. Wholegrain varieties of wheat, barley, oats, rice and maize (corn) have the best nutrient content. Base your main meal and snacks around these low-fat foods for maximum energy and nutrition.

* **Rye** contains many minerals including iron, magnesium and zinc. It is also a good source of energy-releasing B vitamins, folate and vitamin E. Pumpernickel, sourdough and linseed rye breads have a low glycaemic index (GI) value. This means they are digested more slowly than white breads and are therefore excellent for sustaining energy levels. Multi-grain and granary breads are also good choices – try making bread using different grain flours.

* **Wheatgerm** is highly nutritious and rich in magnesium, B vitamins, folate, vitamin E and zinc, all important for energy production. Add the unprocessed form to porridge and breakfast cereals, breads and other bakery products, stews and soups, and any recipe requiring wholemeal flour. You can substitute up to 25% (plus extra fluid) in most recipes to enrich the nutritional content without affecting the end product.

* **Oats** are rich in soluble fibre which slows down the rate of digestion, ensuring a steady release of glucose energy. Add them to breakfast cereals and muesli – oatmeal porridge, in particular, is a very filling, energizing breakfast that will lift your mood.

* **Rice** is versatile, cheap, easy to cook, low in fat and full of carbohydrate energy. Brown rice provides more fibre, minerals and vitamins than white rice. To retain more nutrients, do not rinse the rice before cooking, and steam or microwave it rather than boiling.

FOCUS ON WHEAT-FREE DIETS

* Many foods contain wheat including bread, flour, cakes, biscuits, pasta, sauces and breakfast cereals. If you need a wheat-free diet for health reasons, replace these foods with potatoes, pulses, rice, maize (corn), seeds and nuts. You can use cornflour (cornstarch), potato starch, rice flour or soya flour in recipes to thicken and add bulk.

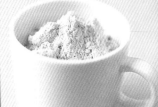

oats

wild rice

corn flour

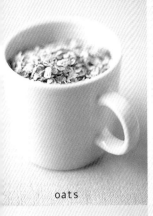

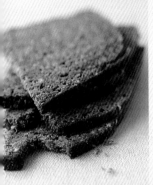

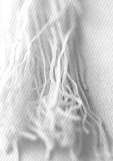

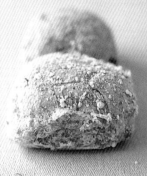

rye bread

tagliolini

wholemeal bread

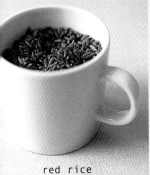

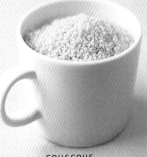

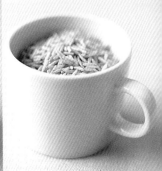

red rice

couscous

brown rice

starchy and root vegetables

These substantial vegetables provide plenty of carbohydrate energy, as well as important vitamins, minerals, antioxidants and fibre.

Starchy vegetables contain high levels of carbohydrate and fibre. Eating potatoes and parsnips cooked whole or in large pieces, particularly with their skin on, rather than in small pieces or mashed, will make them more filling and sustaining. High in essential minerals and vitamins they also boost the body's immune system.

* **Sweet potatoes** are high in starch, vitamin C, beta-carotene and fibre. With a low GI value, they have a longer-lasting effect on energy levels than ordinary potatoes. Use sweet potatoes in soups and casseroles for an evening meal or light supper, or mashed or baked as a vegetable accompaniment instead of ordinary potatoes.

* **Pumpkins and squashes** are low in fat and rich in beta-carotene. Their seeds contain essential omega-6 fatty acids and some carbohydrate and fibre.

* **Beetroot** is low in calories and fat, and is a good source of folate, potassium and flavonoid antioxidants. Its leafy tops are rich in beta-carotene, magnesium, calcium and iron, and can be used in salads or as a cooked vegetable. Add beetroots to salads, or grate them into soups and fish dishes.

* **Globe artichokes** provide fibre and carbohydrate energy, as well as small amounts of most important vitamins and minerals.

* **Carrots** are packed with antioxidants, beta-carotene, fibre and starch. This is one of the only vegetables to have a better nutritional value cooked rather than raw as their tough outer structure prevents some nutrients being absorbed.

FOCUS ON ORGANIC VEGETABLES

* Organic vegetables are grown and processed without the use of synthetic fertilizers or pesticides and artificial additives. Genetically modified (GM) crops are also banned under organic farming standards. While the nutritional value of organic vegetables may be similar to that of non-organic, arguably they are more flavoursome. For varieties to be eaten raw or unpeeled, organic may be the best choice. Make sure the vegetables are really fresh, and use them as soon as possible after purchase as they tend to spoil relatively quickly. You may find the choice of varieties more restricted at certain times of year than with non-organic produce, and there will be a premium on prices, but you should weigh these factors against the possible health benefits.

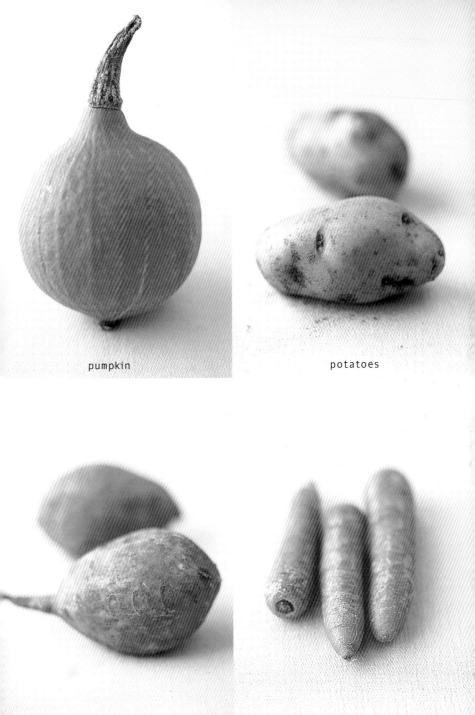

pumpkin

potatoes

sweet potatoes

carrots

herbs, green leafy and salad vegetables

Leafy and salad vegetable groups are packed with vitamins, minerals, antioxidants and fibre. They are also low in calories and fat, making them a very healthy eating option.

* **Dark green leafy vegetables** – such as spinach, broccoli, watercress, kale and pak choi – are highly nutritious, an excellent source of vitamin C and antioxidants and should be eaten regularly for optimal health. Contrary to popular belief, spinach is not rich in iron; it does, however, provide good amounts of potassium, folate and beta-carotene. Use fresh young spinach leaves raw in salads and sandwiches; or use cooked in soups, patés or as a vegetable accompaniment.

* **Lettuce** is low in fat and provides some fibre and antioxidants. This means it provides bulk but few calories, so is a good salad food for weight control. Serve lots of leaves with a vinegar dressing to accompany a carbohydrate-rich meal that includes pasta, potatoes or rice – the vinegar can help to limit the rise in blood sugar by slowing the rate of digestion of the carbohydrate.

* **Red, orange and yellow vegetables,** such as tomatoes, are rich in vitamins, minerals and antioxidants such as beta-carotene. These help boost the body's immune system, protecting against viruses and infections that sap energy and vitality.

* **Red peppers (red capsicums)** are an excellent source of beta-carotene and vitamin C, which facilitates the absorption of iron – try adding red peppers to a beef stir fry for a real iron boost. They are best used raw in salads or dips, stir-fried, or roasted because vitamin C is water soluble and will be destroyed by boiling or cooking in water.

* **Garlic** has a long history of medicinal use, and regular intake may help to reduce blood cholesterol levels. It also provides some calcium, phosphorus, potassium and vitamin C. It is used in a wide range of recipes as a flavour enhancer.

* **Mushrooms** are low in calories and fat, and a good source of folate. Button mushrooms can be eaten raw, chopped into salads to add a nutty taste. Field mushrooms have a stronger flavour – sauté with garlic and serve on rye bread as a snack, or add to soups, pasta and pizzas.

FOCUS ON HERBS

* Most fresh herbs are rich in minerals and vitamins, and also provide fibre and antioxidants. Even though we only eat relatively small amounts of fresh or dried herbs, they can provide a valuable energy boost. Aromatic rosemary, for example, can heighten the senses, stimulating mental activity and combating fatigue while parsley is a good source of iron, vitamin C and fibre.

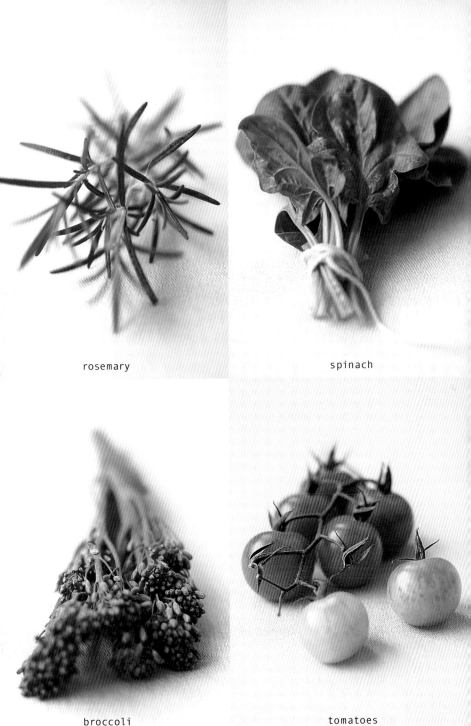

rosemary

spinach

broccoli

tomatoes

fresh fruit

Fruit provides us with fibre and carbohydrate, as well as many of the vitamins and minerals needed for good health and energy production.

You should aim to eat at least three servings of different-coloured fruits every day.

* **Citrus fruits** – oranges, lemons, grapefruit, limes, tangerines, mandarins, satsumas and clementines – are good sources of Vitamin C, a deficiency of which can cause fatigue, loss of appetite and susceptibility to infection.

* **Bananas** are rich in potassium, vitamin B6 and carbohydrate energy. They are best eaten just ripe, for the correct balance of sugar and starch. Use over-ripe bananas to add natural sweetness to dishes, baked in banana bread and muffins, and sliced or mashed in low-fat yoghurt for a nutritious dessert.

* **Apples** are low in calories and fat, and rich in fibre, and fresh apples provide vitamin C and other antioxidants. Apples are ideal snacks and can be used in many savoury and sweet dishes. Add them to muesli, salads, or sauces or bake them.

* **Pears** provide carbohydrate, fibre, potassium and some antioxidants. Use them raw as a snack or in salads, on breakfast cereals, in low-fat yoghurt, or poached in fruit juice for a quick and delicious low-calorie dessert.

* **Plums** are a good source of fibre and antioxidants, such as vitamin C and flavonoids. Use them fresh (or in their dried form, prunes) as an addition to breakfast cereals, low-fat yoghurt and fruit salads, stewed in desserts, and puréed in sauces and marinades.

* **Apricots** (and other exotic yellow and orange fruits such as peaches, mangoes and melons) are good sources of beta-carotene and other antioxidants, as well as potassium and fibre.

* **Berries** are low in calories and fat and rich in vitamin C. A nutritious and refreshing snack on their own, they can be used fresh in the same way as plums and are also wonderful in jams, jellies, pies and crumbles, muffins and cheese-cakes. Dried berries can be used in the same way as other dried fruits.

FOCUS ON NATURAL SWEETENERS

* Fruit contains natural sugars including fructose, which – unlike sucrose, the sugar in table sugar – does not cause a rapid rise in blood sugar levels. Fructose can be used directly by the muscles for energy production, but if eaten in excess it can have a laxative effect. It is much sweeter than sucrose, so you need much less of it to produce the same level of sweetness.

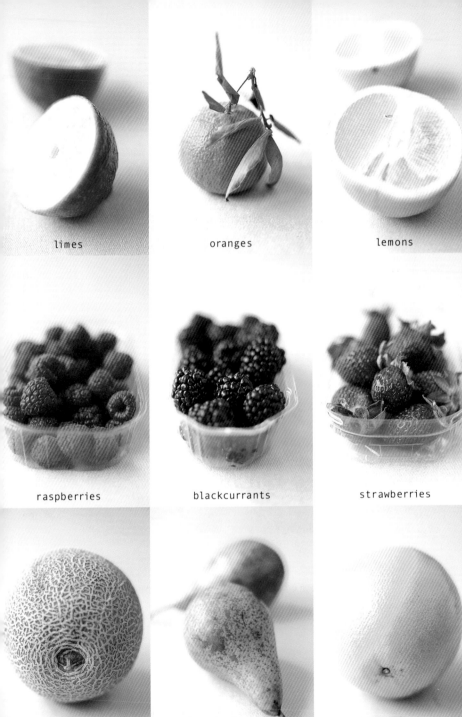

limes

oranges

lemons

raspberries

blackcurrants

strawberries

melon

pears

grapefruit

dried fruits and fruit juices

Dried fruits and fruit juices provide a convenient concentrated source of nutrients for instant energy production as they are higher in natural sugar than fresh fruits.

* **Dates** are a good source of energy, fibre, potassium, magnesium and B vitamins. They also provide some iron and calcium. However, as dates are rich in calories and have a laxative effect, they should not be eaten in excess! Dates also have a high GI value, causing blood sugar levels to rise rapidly, so are best used as a natural sweetener in dishes with other fruits.

* **Dried figs** contain both soluble and insoluble fibre – a small bowlful will have a laxative effect and is a natural remedy for constipation. Dried figs are also rich in energy (calories) and potassium, and are a useful source of calcium, iron and magnesium. Use them to provide natural sweetness in low-fat yogurt, home-made muesli and unsweetened cereals, or in any recipes requiring dried fruit.

* **Sultanas, currants and raisins** are forms of dried grapes. They provide natural sweetness, plenty of calories, fibre and potassium, and some iron and B vitamins. Delicious as a snack or dessert on their own, these versatile ingredients can be used in a wide range of sweet and savoury dishes including muesli, fruit salads, compotes, bakery products, curries, stews, stuffings, sauces, chutneys, risottos and desserts. Rehydrated with fruit juice (or perhaps alcohol), they can be puréed or used whole for extra sweetness and flavour in low-fat, sugar-free mousses, fools, yoghurts and sorbets.

* **Fruit juices** can provide a quick boost to blood sugar, energy and nutrient levels. As the structure of the fruit is already broken down in juice, sugars and nutrients are immediately available to the body for energy production. Juices are also an excellent source of vitamin C and antioxidants, boosting the immune system and iron absorption. Drink juice alone or with water to maintain body fluid levels. One serving of fruit juice (as part of a balanced diet) is 120ml (4fl oz).

FOCUS ON DRIED FRUITS

* You can buy almost any type of fruit in dried form. Dried fruits provide a concentrated source of nutrients – in particular fibre, sugar energy, iron and potassium – and their high sugar content means that they last far longer than fresh fruits. Being such a rich source of energy, dried fruits are also much higher in calories than their fresh equivalents, so keep an eye on your intake if you are trying to control your weight.

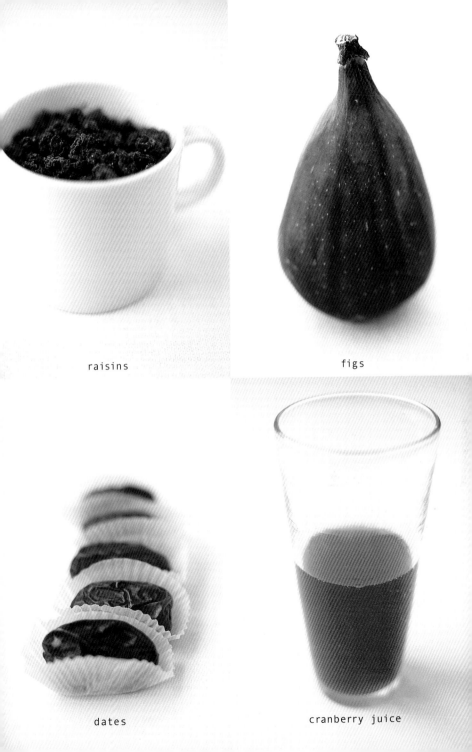

raisins

figs

dates

cranberry juice

Rich in potassium, phosphorus, iron and iodine, beta-carotene, vitamin E and B vitamins.

rye cakes with fresh fruit and yoghurt
Prep time: 10 minutes, cooking time: about 20 minutes, serves 4

125g (4½oz) rye flour or combination of rye and buckwheat flours
1 heaped teaspoon baking powder
Pinch of salt
1 tablespoon brown or unrefined brown sugar
2 eggs
250g (9oz) low-fat bio (natural) yoghurt
25g (1oz) butter or 1 tablespoon sunflower oil
Sliced bananas or fruit compote
(see page 50), to serve
Low-fat bio (natural) yoghurt, to serve
Maple syrup or honey, to serve (optional)

Sift the flour, baking powder, salt and sugar in a large bowl. Beat the eggs in another bowl and stir in the yoghurt. Stir the egg mixture into the dry ingredients until well combined and smooth.

Heat the butter or oil in a frying pan over a medium-high heat. Drop about 1 tablespoon of the batter into the frying pan, spreading it out to make small but thick cakes about 6cm (2½oz) across. Cook for 1 minute on either side.

Remove and place on warm plates, allowing about 3 cakes per person. Serve immediately with sliced banana or fruit compote, a dollop of yoghurt, and maple syrup or honey if using.
PER SERVING: 224kcals/950kJ 9g protein 4g fat 39g carbohydrate 4g fibre

> Served with fruit, this dish provides a wide enough range of nutrients to make it a complete meal in itself. Being high in carbohydrates, it is an ideal way to start the day and is also a quick and nourishing dish to make at any time when your energy levels are flagging. The cakes are suitable for a wheat-free diet – use buckwheat and gluten-free baking powder for a gluten-free diet. Bio yogurt is suitable for those with digestive problems; use live soya-, goat's- or sheep's-milk yoghurt for a diet free of cow's milk.

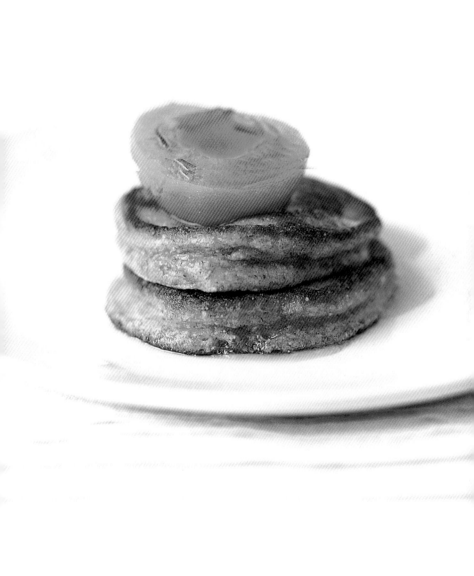

An excellent source of potassium, beta-carotene and vitamin C.

fruit salad with ginger and chinese five spice

Prep time: 15 minutes, cooking time: nil, serves 4.

½ ripe cantaloupe (rockmelon) or charantais melon

1 large ripe mango

1 large ripe papaya (pawpaw)

1 kiwi

1 pomegranate (optional)

1 piece of stem ginger, finely chopped

Pinch of Chinese five spice (optional)

1 tablespoon syrup from the stem ginger

2 teaspoons lime juice

Remove the skin from the cantaloupe (rockmelon), cut into thin wedges and then cut each wedge in half. Cut the 2 mango cheeks from either side of the stone, peel and cut into thin slices.

Cut the papaya (pawpaw) in half, remove the seeds and peel, then slice thinly and cut each slice in half. Peel the kiwi and cut into round slices. Cut the pomegranate in half if using, and remove the small juicy seeds, discarding any white pith.

Place the fruit in a bowl or on a plate, scatter over the pomegranate seeds, ginger, and Chinese five spice if using. Pour over the ginger syrup and lime juice, and serve immediately.

Note: A variety of fruits can be used, but tropical fruits work best with the spices. If you cannot find Chinese five spice, it can be omitted.

PER SERVING: 90kcals/385kJ 1g protein trace of fat 22g carbohydrate 3g fibre

---

This colourful dish is great for lifting your mood – especially on a dark winter morning when sunlight is scarce. It is also brilliant for the immune system, boosting antioxidants and vitamin C levels to protect cells and help ward off winter colds and flus. The spices are warming and ginger is good for the digestive system, making it ideal for those with food intolerances or digestive problems. Serve the fruit salad with yoghurt, porridge or muesli to provide a nutritious breakfast, or as a snack at any time of the day to boost flagging blood sugar levels.

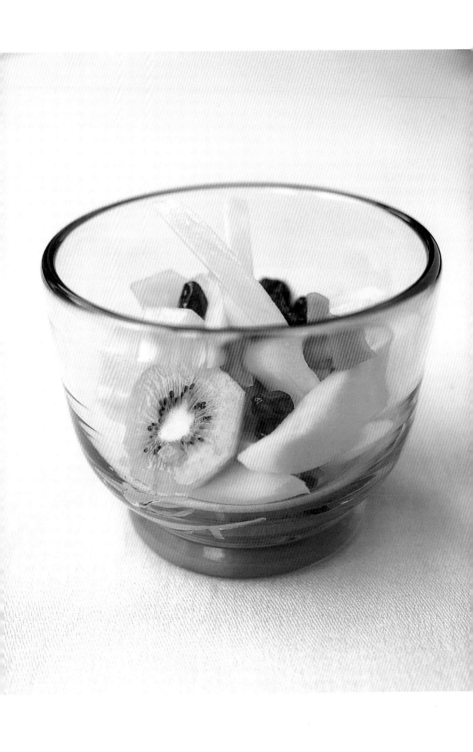

Rich in a range of minerals, as well as vitamin E
and B vitamins, especially folate.

easy one-rise, multi-grain bread

Prep time: 15 minutes, resting time: 1 hour, cooking time: 30 minutes, makes 2 loaves
each providing approximately 10 thick slices

500g (1lb 2oz) granary (wholegrain) or
wholemeal flour
200g (7oz) rye flour
100g (3½ oz) rolled whole oats
75g (2¾ oz) pumpkin seeds
15g (½ oz) sesame seeds
15g (½ oz) mustard or poppy seeds
2 heaped teaspoons salt

3 teaspoons dried yeast or 1½ sachets
easy active yeast
2 teaspoons maple syrup or honey
500ml (18 fl oz) warm water
2 tablespoons milk or water, for glazing
25g (1oz) rolled whole oats, for decorating
25g (1oz) pumpkin seeds, for decorating

Place all the dry ingredients in a large bowl, or in a food mixer with a bread hook. Add the
maple syrup or honey and water and mix until the mixture is amalgamated, then knead for
about 5–10 minutes. If using loaf tins, lightly grease 2 x 1kg (2lb) tins with butter or oil.

Divide the dough in half and place in the tins. Alternatively, shape the dough into 2 large
round balls and place on a greased oven tray, with at least 20cm (8in) between them.
Glaze the bread with the milk or water and decorate with the extra oats and pumpkin seeds.
Leave the bread to rise near the oven for at least 1 hour until double in size. (As long as
the kitchen is not draughty, leave the bread uncovered to rise slowly rather than too fast in
too warm a place.) Preheat the oven to 200°C (400°F/Gas 6). When the bread is ready,
place in the oven and cook for about 30 minutes until golden brown. Remove the bread
from the oven and tap the back: when cooked, it should sound hollow. Leave to cool for at
least 30 minutes before slicing. The bread can be frozen successfully.

PER SERVING: 150kcals/650kJ 5g protein 3g fat (mainly mono-and polyunsaturated)
27g carbohydrate 4g fibre

This bread is an excellent source of carbohydrate to sustain blood sugar levels and provide the
essential minerals and B vitamins for energy production. A couple of slices make an ideal high-
carbohydrate, low-fat snack at any time of the day with low-fat spread – especially useful for
active people or as a bedtime snack. Top with homemade hummus and fresh parsley or eggs and
tomatoes to make a high-protein complete snack for earlier in the day.

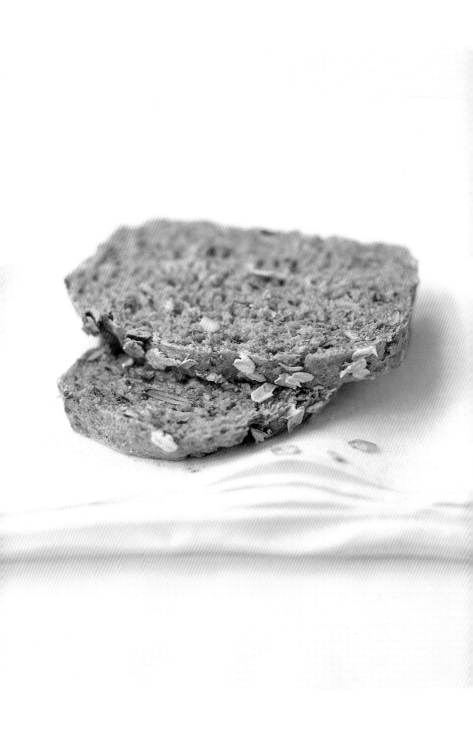

Provides potassium, phosphorus, iron and calcium,
as well as B vitamins, including folate.

cherry muffins with buckwheat

Prep time: 10 minutes, cooking time: 20 minutes, makes 8–10 large muffins

200g (7oz) plain flour

50g (1¾ oz) buckwheat or wholemeal flour

100g (3½ oz) unrefined caster sugar

½ teaspoon salt

1 teaspoon ground cinnamon

1 heaped teaspoon baking powder

50g (1¾ oz) almonds, roughly chopped
and toasted

2 eggs

200ml (7fl oz) buttermilk or low-fat bio
(natural) yoghurt

2 tablespoons sunflower or nut oil

½ teaspoon vanilla extract

150g (5½ oz) drained cherries from a jar or
fresh pitted cherries, quartered

Icing sugar, for dusting (optional)

Preheat the oven to 190°C (375°F/Gas 5) and lightly grease a tray of 8 muffin cups (½ cup capacity) or use paper liners.

Place the flours, sugar, salt, cinnamon, baking powder and chopped almonds in a mixing bowl. Beat the eggs in another bowl and stir in the buttermilk or yoghurt, oil, vanilla and cherries. Stir the egg mixture into the dry ingredients until just combined.

For good, fluffy muffins, fill the muffin cups until level with the top. Bake for 20 minutes, or until the tops are lightly browned and a skewer inserted in the middle of a muffin comes out clean. Cool on a wire rack and dust with icing sugar if using.

Note: Other soft fruit such as raspberries or blueberries can be substituted.

**PER MUFFIN: 210 kcals/880 kJ 6.5g protein 6g fat (mainly mono-and polyunsaturated)
35g carbohydrate 2g fibre**

These muffins are excellent carbohydrate providers to sustain blood sugar levels through-out the morning or as a snack at any time of the day. They are also good for supper to prevent waking from hunger in the night. Providing a range of minerals and B vitamins, these muffins are good for energy production, healthy immunity and thyroid function.

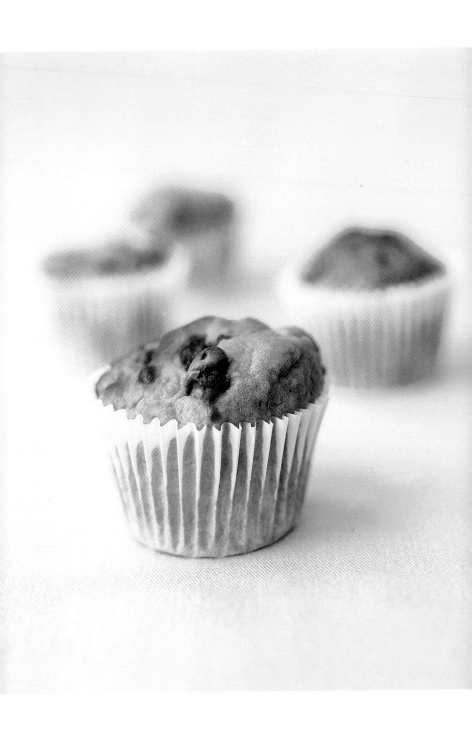

Rich in potassium, calcium, magnesium, phosphorus, iron.
Also a good source of vitamin C, beta-carotene and folate.

fruit compote

Prep time: 15 minutes, cooking time: 10 minutes, serves 4

75 g (2¾ oz) dried apricots, quartered
75 g (2¾ oz) dried peaches or mango, quartered
75 g (2¾ oz) dried cherries or cranberries
50 g (1¾ oz) stoned dates, cut in half

25 g (1oz) raisins or currants
250 ml (9fl oz) apple juice or water
1 small cinnamon stick
½ vanilla pod, split
2 pieces of stem ginger, finely chopped

Place the dried fruits in a saucepan and add the apple juice or water, cinnamon stick and vanilla pod. Bring to the boil, cover and simmer gently for 10 minutes.

Add the ginger off the heat and leave to cool. Transfer to a bowl or airtight container, cover and refrigerate, where it will last for at least a week. Serve a large spoonful on top of some yogurt or good-quality muesli for a nourishing breakfast.

PER SERVING: 150kcals/650kJ 2g protein trace of fat 38g carbohydrate 7g fibre

This colourful dish is an excellent carbohydrate, vitamin and mineral provider. You can buy organic dried fruit or pre-soak the fruit in alcohol, warm water or fruit juice and rinse to remove traces of the sulphites and mineral oils used to preserve them. Serve as suggested, or on its own with yoghurt for a wheat-/gluten-free diet.

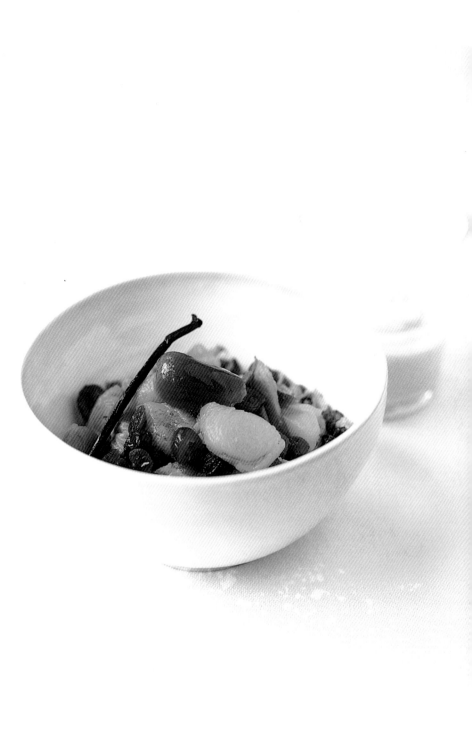

Provides plenty of slow-release carbohydrates.

banana and honey smoothie

Prep time: under 10 minutes, serves 1

1 ripe banana
250 ml (9 fl oz) soya or semi-skimmed milk
Dash of honey or maple syrup
1 tablespoon low-fat bio (natural) yoghurt
(optional)

Place the banana and soya or semi-skimmed milk in a blender. Add the honey or maple syrup and yoghurt if using. Blend until frothy.
   Note: A variety of soft fresh fruits and rehydrated dried fruits can be substituted for the banana.
PER SERVING: 180kcals/751kJ 8g protein 5g fat 27g carbohydrate

Especially rich in potassium and vitamin C.

cranberry and grapefruit drink

Prep time: under 5 minutes, serves 1

100 ml (3½ fl oz) cranberry juice
100 ml (3½ fl oz) grapefruit juice, freshly squeezed

Mix together equal quantities of cranberry juice and freshly squeezed grapefruit juice, for a drink that is full of vitamins.
PER SERVING: 60kcals/280kJ 16g carbohydrate

Relaxing bedtime drink to enhance sleep.

mint tea

Prep time: under 5 minutes, serves 1

Small bunch of fresh mint leaves
200 ml (7 fl oz) boiling water

Place the mint leaves in the bottom of a mug or in a teapot and pour boiling water over them. Leave to infuse for 1 minute and drink while still hot. Traditionally, Moroccans would add sugar, but this is not necessary.
   Note: Lemon verbena or fresh chamomile buds can be infused in the same way.
PER SERVING: Calorie and fat free

Very refreshing first thing in the morning.

hot water and lemon

Prep time: under 5 minutes, serves 1

Lemon peel
200 ml (7 fl oz) boiling water

For a simple yet very pleasant-tasting drink, cut a piece of lemon peel, place it in a mug and pour boiling water over it. This drink is especialy good if you want to avoid caffeinated drinks altogether but find other herbal infusions too strong tasting.
PER SERVING: Calorie and fat free

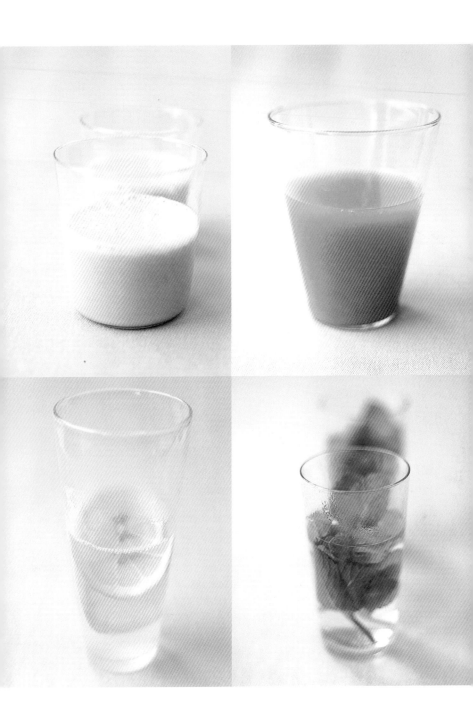

ready-made snacks

A selection of ideas for foods to buy that are ready prepared but still healthy – eat them when you are in a hurry, on the move or as nutritious snacks at any time.

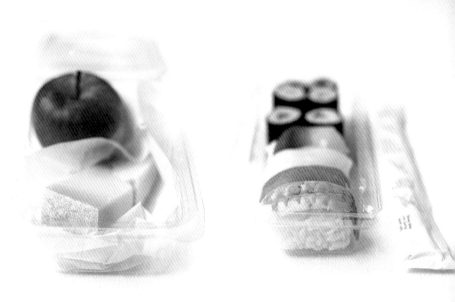

Good source of calcium, fibre and vitamin C.

apple and cheese

The simplest of high-protein snacks. Choose a delicious crunchy organic apple and a tasty piece of mature cheddar, or taleggio. No preparation and lots of nutrients. Use low-fat cheese to reduce the calories and fat.

PER SERVING (apple and 1oz/25g mature hard cheese): 150 kcals/620 kJ 7g protein 9g fat 12g carbohydrate 2g fibre

Good source of B vitamins and minerals.

sushi box

Sushi is now widely available in high street stores and sandwich shops, and makes an ideal snack food. The nori is full of nutrients, the rice provides carbohydrate and the fish is rich in protein, with tuna and salmon being good sources of essential fatty acids.

PER 100g (3½ oz) SERVING (half oily fish, half rice): less than 200 kcals/840 kJ 15g protein 16g carbohydrate 5g fat

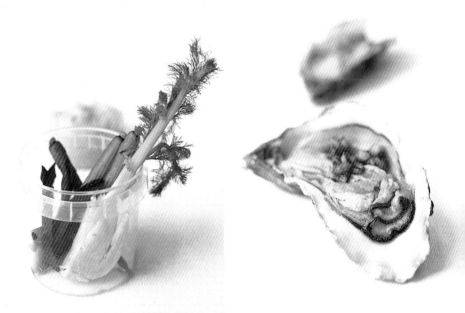

Rich in a range of vitamins and minerals.

Rich in vitamin B12, zinc, selenium and iodine.

hummus with raw vegetables

Full of chickpeas and sesame seeds, hummus makes a nutritious, energy-boosting snack. Eat it with crunchy raw vegetables such as carrot, cauliflower and pepper (capsicum) to keep hunger at bay.

PER 120g (4¼oz) SERVING (half vegetables, half hummus): 130 kcals/ 550kJ 6g protein 8g fat

oysters

Although not usually regarded as a snack food, oysters are nevertheless quick to eat, low in fat and packed full of zinc .

PER 100g (3½oz) SERVING (in shells): 26kcals/110kJ 5g protein less than 1g fat

fast foods

Whether you need a morning boost, a relaxing bedtime snack, or to prevent a mid-afternoon dip, these quick-fix foods will keep blood sugar and energy levels constant.

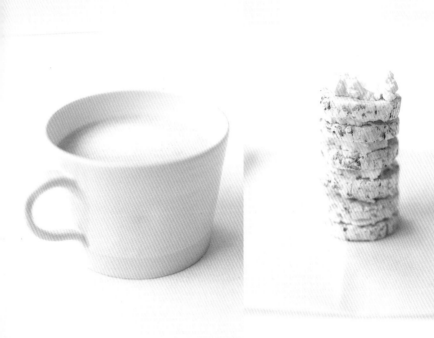

An excellent source of minerals and vitamins.

Rich in niacin and carbohydrate.

malted drinks

Drinking a cup of malted milk, full of nutrients, is a good way to help you get to sleep at night. Hot milk and honey is another simple but satisfying late-night drink that would also be relaxing at any time of the day.

PER SERVING (mug): 160 kcals/690 kJ 8g protein 4g fat 26g carbohydrate

rice cakes

Rice cakes are a good snack choice if you have a wheat intolerance. Top with tahini (sesame spread) for a high calcium savoury snack, or try them with cheese or fruit.

PER SERVING (6 mini rice cakes): 44kcals/184kJ 10g carbohydrate 1g protein less than 1g fat 1g fibre

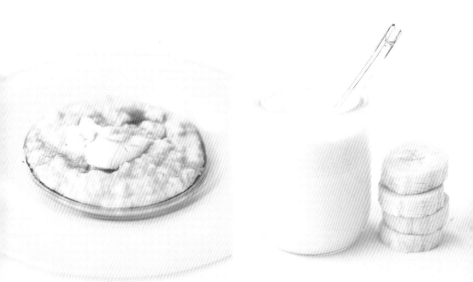

Carbohydrate-boosting snack or breakfast.

Full of zinc and potassium.

porridge

Oats are a great source of carbohydrate and fibre. They are, of course, wheat free and widely available in snacks such as flapjacks, oatcake biscuits or cereal bars. Classic porridge with a dollop of yoghurt and honey or maple syrup is the perfect way to start the day.

PER SERVING (bowl of porridge): 110 kcals/ 470 kJ 4 g protein 20 g carbohydrate 2 g fat 1 g fibre

yoghurt with banana and maple syrup

For a filling snack, mix low-fat bio (natural) yoghurt with slices of banana – add a dash of maple syrup as an optional treat.

PER SERVING (small 125g/4oz pot of low-fat yoghurt, 1 medium banana and 1 teaspoon maple syrup): 170 kcals/ 710 kJ 7 g protein 32 g carbohydrate 1 g fat 3 g fibre

Rich in minerals, vitamins E and C, and B vitamins.

chickpea pancakes with prawns and coconut chutney

Prep time: 30 minutes, cooking time: 10 minutes, serves 4

300g (10½oz) large raw tiger prawns, peeled
1 tablespoon sunflower oil
1 heaped tablespoon coarsely chopped fresh coriander, plus extra to serve
3 spring onions, trimmed and finely sliced at an angle
2 large tomatoes, diced
Juice of ½ lime, plus wedges to serve
Pancakes:
200g (7oz) chickpea flour
½ large red or green chilli, finely chopped
2 cloves garlic, finely chopped
2 heaped tablespoons coarsely chopped fresh coriander
100g (3½oz) low-fat bio (natural) yoghurt
Large pinch of salt

250ml (9fl oz) water
Sunflower oil, for frying
Coconut chutney:
50g (1¾oz) unsweetened desiccated coconut
125ml (4floz) boiling water
2 heaped tablespoons chopped fresh ginger
1 clove garlic, chopped
½ large red or green chilli, chopped
1 teaspoon fennel seeds (optional)
1 tablespoon sunflower oil
1 level tablespoon black mustard seeds (optional)
1 tablespoon low-fat bio (natural) yoghurt
1 heaped tablespoon coarsely chopped fresh coriander
Salt, to taste

For the pancakes, place the chickpea flour in a bowl and add the chilli, garlic, coriander, yoghurt and salt. Pour in the water and mix to form a thick batter without lumps. Set aside.

To make the chutney, combine the coconut with the boiling water and mix well. Puree the ginger, garlic, chilli and fennel seeds if using, in a pestle and mortar or small blender. Gently heat the oil with the mustard seeds if using, and cover with a lid. Once the seeds have started popping, add the spices and cook gently for 1 minute, stirring continuously. Remove from the heat and add the coconut. Once cooled, add the yoghurt, coriander and salt to taste.

Heat a frying pan (about 25cm/10in across) and wipe with a kitchen towel drenched in sunflower oil. Pour in enough chickpea batter to just cover the width of the frying pan, spreading out as it cooks. Cook the pancake for 3 minutes on each side, until lightly browned. Set aside on a plate in a warm oven until all four pancakes have been cooked.

To cook the prawns, heat the pan over a high heat, add the oil and cook the prawns for about 1 minute, until they change colour. Remove from the heat and add the coriander, spring onions, tomatoes and lime juice. Serve the pancakes with the prawns, chutney and lime wedges.

PER SERVING: 400kcals/1660kJ 30g protein 18g fat 30g carbohydrate 10g fibre

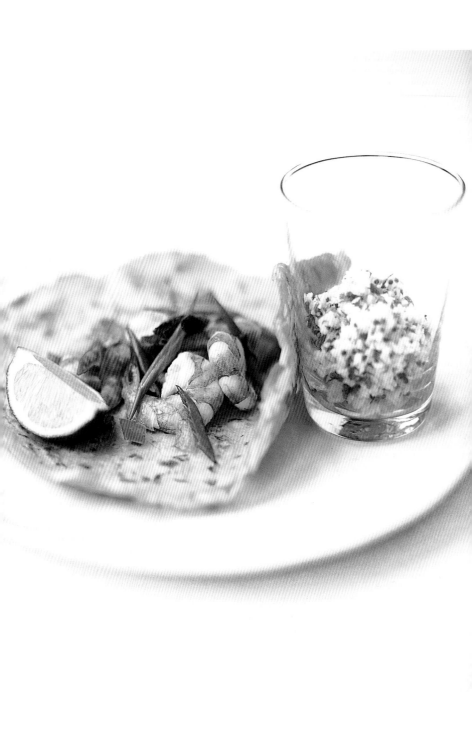

Provides a good range of important minerals plus
beta-carotene, vitamins E and C, and B vitamins.

chinese beef stir fry with rice noodles and vegetables

Prep time: 20 minutes, cooking time: 6 minutes, serves 4

2 medium carrots, peeled, cut in half lengthways and thinly sliced

1 red pepper (capsicum), quartered, deseeded
and thinly sliced

100g (3½oz) mangetout (snowpeas) or sugar
snap peas, finely sliced at an angle

4 spring onions, trimmed and sliced

200g (7oz) rice noodles (vermicelli or thick style)

2 heaped tablespoons chopped fresh ginger

2 large cloves garlic, finely chopped

2 tablespoons sesame oil

3 tablespoons sunflower oil

2 medium-sized sirloin steaks or 500g
(1lb 2oz) beef fillet, cut into strips

1 tablespoon black bean sauce

1 tablespoon oyster or soy sauce

1 tablespoon hoisin sauce or 1 teaspoon
Chinese five spice

1 tablespoon chilli sauce or ½ large chilli,
finely chopped

4 tablespoons chicken stock or water

4 heaped tablespoons coarsely chopped fresh
coriander, stalks included

Prepare all the vegetables before cooking, as the cooking time is so brief. Soak the noodles in
hot water, immersing them completely. Mix well to break up the noodles and prevent them
sticking together. Leave to soften, then drain just before cooking.

Place the ginger and garlic in a wok. Add the sesame oil and 2 tablespoons of the sunflower
oil and turn the heat to high. Cook for about 1 minute until the wok is hot. Add the vegetables
and cook for 2 minutes, stirring frequently, until tender-crisp. Transfer the vegetables to a bowl.

Heat the remaining sunflower oil in the wok, then add the beef. Cook for about 1 minute,
turning the meat over until both sides are just browned. Quickly add the black bean sauce,
oyster or soy sauce, hoisin sauce or five spice, and chilli sauce or chopped chilli, mix briefly,
and then add the meat to the vegetables, leaving behind as much liquid as possible.

Add the drained noodles and the stock or water to the wok, cooking for about 1–2 minutes
until the noodles are soft and tender. Finally, add the beef, vegetables and coriander to the wok
and stir off the heat until well mixed. Serve immediately.

Note: Use very lean beef in this recipe to keep down the fat content. If you cannot find
sesame oil, substitute sunflower oil.

PER SERVING: 500 kcals/2080kJ 34g protein 24g fat 40g carbohydrate 3g fibre

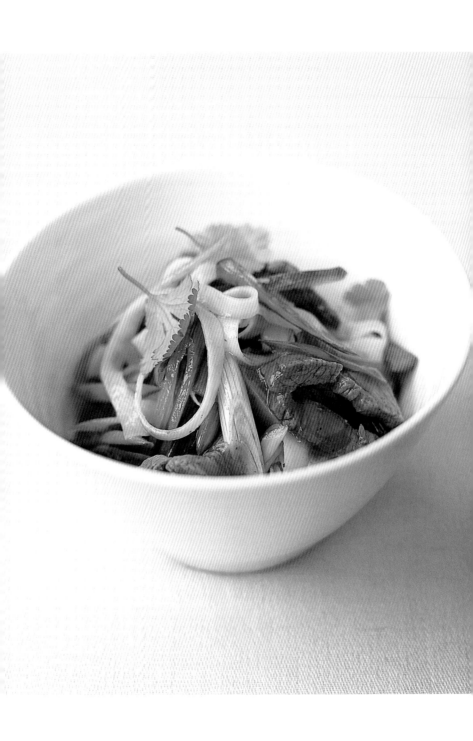

Very rich in iron, vitamin A and B vitamins, particularly B12 and folate.

pan-fried calves' liver
Prep time: 5 minutes, cooking time: 15 minutes, serves 2

2 tablespoons extra-virgin olive oil	12 sage leaves
1 medium red onion, halved and thinly sliced	2 tablespoons balsamic vinegar
1 large clove garlic, thinly sliced	Salt and pepper, to taste
250g (9oz) calves' liver, thinly sliced and trimmed	creamed potatoes or polenta, to serve

Pour the olive oil into a large frying pan and gently cook the onion and garlic for about 10 minutes until soft and lightly caramelized. Push the onion mixture to the side of the pan and increase the heat to high. Lay the liver flat in the pan with the sage and sear each side for about 30 seconds to 1 minute. Quickly add the balsamic vinegar and remove from the heat. Season with salt and pepper and remove the liver, placing it on top of some creamed potatoes or polenta. If the vinegar is too reduced, add a dash of water and place back on the heat, stirring the sediment and onion mixture at the base of the pan until it is reduced to a thick sauce. Taste for seasoning, then pour the onion and vinegar mixture over the liver and serve immediately.
PER SERVING: 300 kcals/1275 kJ 26g protein 20g fat 6g carbohydrate 13.8mg iron

Serve the liver with creamed potatoes, as suggested, and lightly steamed green beans or stir-fried colourful vegetables such as courgettes (zucchini), mixed peppers (capsicums), carrots and fennel leaves. Add a glass of fruit juice for a balanced main meal containing all the essential nutrients for energy production and well-being. This dish is an excellent source of iron – providing all your daily requirement – folate and B12, for healthy blood production and to top up your body stores. The sage and garlic also have a positive effect on the immune system. Especially good for people with or prone to anaemia, those with a small appetite or who are recovering from an illness. This dish is not suitable for pregnant women or those trying to conceive.

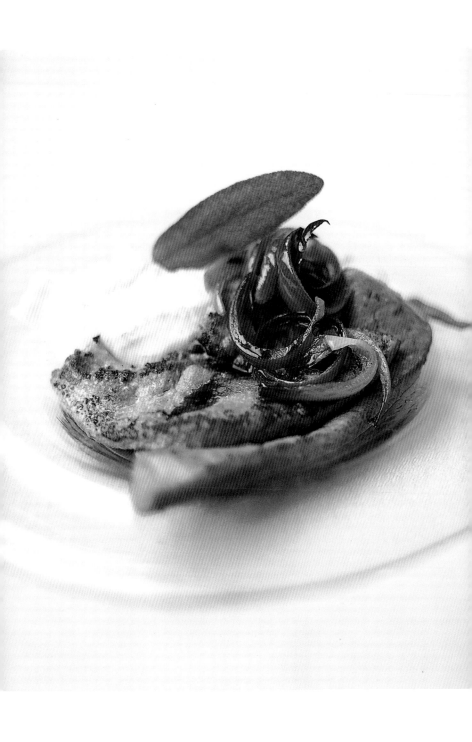

Low in fat and calories; rich in carbohydrate, iron calcium, beta-carotene, vitamin E and B vitamins.

tandoori tofu kebabs

Prep time: 20 minutes, marinating time: 4 hours, cooking time: 15 minutes, serves 4

4 large wooden or metal skewers
400g (14oz) firm good-quality tofu
175g (6oz) low-fat bio (natural) yoghurt
1 heaped teaspoon fresh garam masala, or good pinch each of ground cumin, coriander, cardamom and cinnamon

1 heaped teaspoon chickpea flour or cornflour (cornstarch)
1 heaped teaspoon paprika
1 tablespoon finely chopped fresh ginger
1 large clove garlic, finely chopped
Salt, to taste
Lime or lemon wedges, to serve

If using wooden skewers, soak them in water for 10 minutes to prevent burning. Remove the tofu from the water in which it is stored and drain well on several sheets of kitchen towel for about 15 minutes. Cut into 2.5cm (1in) cubes.

Mix the yoghurt with the garam masala or other spices, flour, paprika, ginger and garlic. Season well with salt and add the tofu cubes. Mix gently to prevent the tofu from breaking up, and leave to marinate in the fridge for about 4 hours or overnight.

Heat the grill to hot and thread the tofu onto four skewers, making sure the tofu is well covered with the yoghurt mixture. Place the kebabs on a greased piece of kitchen foil and grill for about 15 minutes, turning until the tofu is browned all over. Serve the kebabs with a wedge of lime or lemon, accompanied by basmati rice cooked with a pinch of saffron and a few cardamom pods.

PER SERVING: 225 kcal/945 kJ 13g protein 5g fat 33g carbohydrate 2g fibre

Suitable for vegetarians and those on a wheat-free diet, this dish could be adapted for a cow's milk-free diet if goat's-milk or soya yoghurt is used. It is an excellent source of calcium and antioxidants, low in fat and calories and high in carbohydrates, making it an ideal evening meal or supper dish. Serve with fruit juice to boost the vitamin C content.

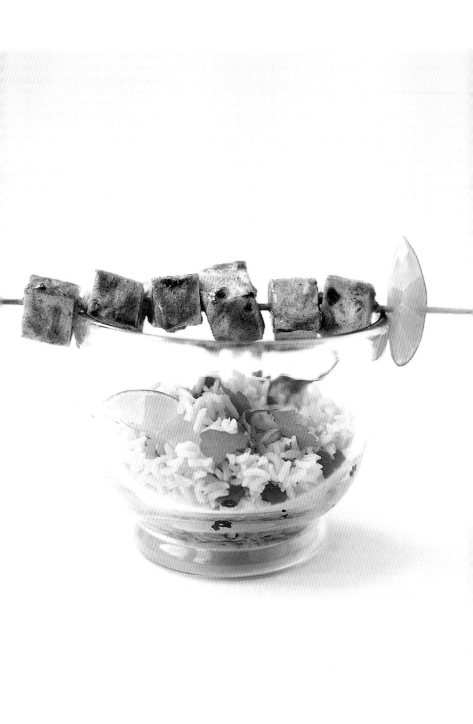

Rich in iron, potassium, phosphorus, zinc, vitamins C and E, and B vitamins.

lamb cutlets with flageolet beans

Prep time: 10 minutes, cooking time: 1 hour, serves 4

250g (9oz) dried flageolet beans (see note)
6 medium-sized vine-ripened tomatoes
(450g/1lb)
4 tablespoons fresh pesto or herb mixture
(see note)
2 whole cloves garlic

1 whole red chilli, fresh or dried (optional)
1 tablespoon extra-virgin olive oil
Salt and pepper, to taste
8 lamb cutlets
2 tablespoons fresh flat-leaf parsley, to serve

If using dried beans, soak in cold water for 6 hours or overnight. Preheat the oven to 200°C (400°F/Gas 6). Cut the tomatoes across the equator and place cut side up on an oiled oven tray or gratin dish. Spoon 1 teaspoon of pesto or herb mixture on top of each tomato. Roast for 40 minutes to 1 hour until very soft and the juices have reduced. While the tomatoes are cooking, drain the beans, place in a saucepan and cover with water. Bring to the boil, skimming any foam that rises to the surface of the water (this helps to avoid the possibility of flatulence often associated with pulses). Add the garlic, chilli if using, and olive oil. Simmer gently until tender – about 40 minutes to 1 hour, depending on how fresh the beans are. Do not add salt to the beans while cooking, as this will toughen them. Drain and place in a bowl. Once the tomatoes are cooked, cut into quarters and add to the beans. Season to taste with salt and pepper, and serve hot or at room temperature. Grill or barbecue the lamb cutlets, cooking for about 3–5 minutes on each side. Serve on top of the bean mixture; sprinkle the parsley on top.

Note: Cannellini beans may be substituted for the flageolet beans. Use a 400g (14oz) can of beans, rinsed, drained, and mixed with 1 crushed garlic clove, ½ large chopped chilli and 1 tablespoon extra-virgin olive oil in place of the dried beans if you like. Instead of fresh pesto, you can use 4 tablespoons chopped fresh basil or parsley, mixed with 1 finely chopped garlic clove and 2 tablespoons extra-virgin olive oil.

PER SERVING: 540 kcals/2260 kJ 30g protein 40g fat 17g carbohydrate 5g fibre

The beans and lamb give this dish its high protein and iron content. The vitamin C provided by the tomatoes and parsley will help with the absorption of iron, making it ideal for topping up stores for healthy blood production and to combat anaemia. The basil, parsley and garlic are also good for the immune system. Serve with garlic bread or potatoes to increase carbohydrate levels for a supper dish, or finish with a carbohydrate-rich dessert for a balanced main meal.

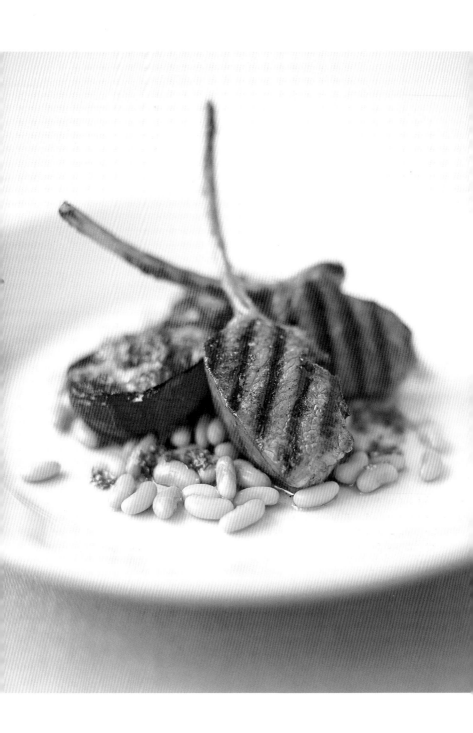

Rich in potassium, phosphorus, iron, iodine, selenium,
beta-carotene and folate. Also high in carbohydrate,
protein and essential fatty acids.

chicken with prunes and bacon

Prep time: 15 minutes, cooking time: 50–65 minutes, serves 4

2 tablespoons olive oil
8 skinned boneless chicken thighs
1 medium onion, quartered and sliced
4 rashers smoked streaky bacon or pancetta, chopped
2 cloves garlic, sliced
1 tablespoon chopped fresh rosemary or thyme
2 medium-sized carrots, cut in half lengthways, then into thick slices

1 piece of stem ginger, chopped, or 1 tablespoon chopped fresh ginger
200g (7oz) Agen or ready-to-eat prunes, stoned and cut in half
350ml (12fl oz) red wine or chicken stock
150ml (5fl oz) cold water mixed with 1 tablespoon cornflour (cornstarch)
Salt and pepper, to taste

Heat the olive oil in a large flameproof casserole or heavy-based saucepan with a lid. Add the chicken and cook over a medium-high heat until lightly browned. Remove from the pan and set aside. Add the onion and bacon or pancetta to the pan and cook over a medium heat for about 10 minutes, stirring regularly and scraping the base of the pan to dislodge any tasty sediment. Once the onion is soft and the bacon browned, add the garlic, rosemary or thyme, carrots and ginger, and cook for a further 2 minutes. Pour in the prunes and the wine or stock, bring to the boil and cook for 1 minute more. Add the cornflour (cornstarch) mixture, bring back to the boil and add the chicken. Season with salt and pepper. Reduce the heat to low, cover with the lid and cook for about 30 minutes until the chicken is cooked. Serve with brown basmati rice flavoured with a pinch of saffron, or mashed sweet or plain potatoes.

Note: You can use chicken thighs on the bone for this dish if preferred – increase the cooking time to 45 minutes.

PER SERVING: 370kcals/1550kJ 29g protein 15g fat 27g carbohydrate 7g fibre

Suitable for wheat- and dairy-free diets, this dish provides plenty of protein and carbohydrate, with useful fibre to maintain a healthy digestive system. The olive oil provides essential fatty acids and the carrots protective antioxidants and beta-carotene. Try using cranberry juice instead of wine to increase antioxidant levels, boost the immune system and enhance iron absorption. Serve with potatoes as suggested to add more carbohydrate for an evening meal, or on its own with fruit or fruit juice for a high-protein, balanced midday meal.

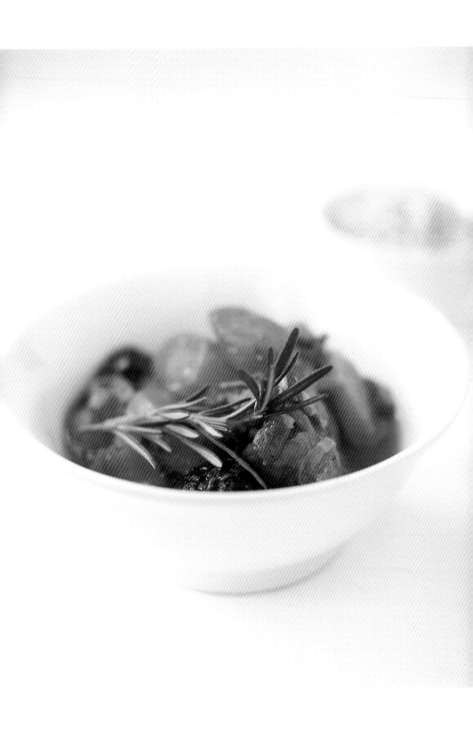

Provides plenty of protein and useful amounts of iron, iodine, selenium and vitamin B12.

scallops wrapped in bacon

Prep time: 15 minutes, cooking time: 8–10 minutes, serves 4

12 thin rashers smoked streaky bacon
12 large scallops, cleaned and drained
4 long thick sturdy sprigs of rosemary

Salt and pepper, to taste
Lemon wedges, to serve

Lay a bacon rasher out flat with a scallop at the bottom, then roll up the bacon at a slight angle so that the scallop is completely covered. Repeat with the remaining bacon and scallops. Trim the rosemary springs to about 18cm (7in) long. Thread three scallops onto each rosemary sprig, starting at the stem end so that the leaves go through easily. Place on a plate and repeat with the rest of the scallops and rosemary. Season with salt and pepper. Heat a griddle (char grill) or frying pan and cook the scallops over a medium-high heat for 8–10 minutes, turning them over until the bacon is golden brown and the scallops just firm and cooked. Serve immediately with a wedge of lemon, accompanied by grilled courgettes (zucchini) or cooked spinach, and rice or potatoes.

Note: Substitute 12 chunks of monkfish for the scallops if you like. If you do not have suitable rosemary sprigs, wooden or metal skewers can be used instead. Be sure to soak the wooden skewers in cold water for 10 minutes beforehand. The scallops can be cooked under the grill if you like.

PER SERVING: 170 kcals/710 kJ 16g protein 12g fat less than 1g carbohydrate

This high-protein, low-fat, low-calorie dish will provide a balanced and nutritious evening meal if served as suggested with rice or potatoes to provide carbohydrate. Serve with roasted vegetables such as peppers (capsicums), tomatoes and garlic to add colour, vitamin C and anti-oxidants to boost the immune system, protect body cells and lift your mood after a tiring day.

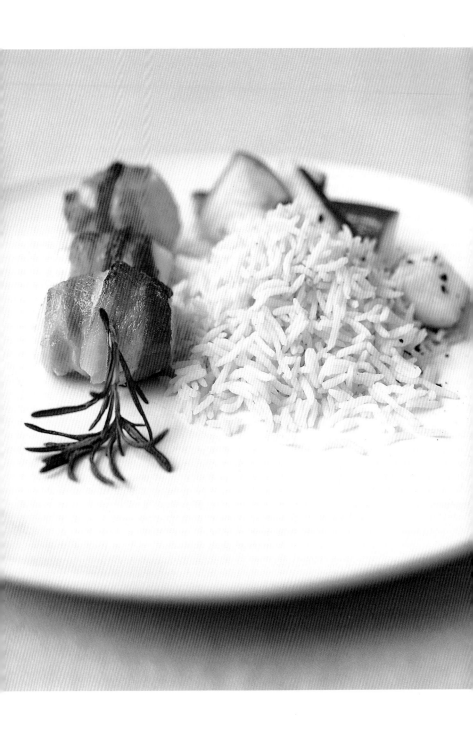

Contains potassium, calcium, phosphorus, iron, zinc, selenium, iodine, beta-carotene, vitamins C and E, and B vitamins.

smoked cod with harissa, leeks and spinach

Prep time: 10 minutes, cooking time: 30 minutes, serves 2

1 tablespoon extra-virgin olive oil
2 large leeks, trimmed, halved and thinly sliced
1 clove garlic, thinly sliced
salt and pepper, to taste
1 tablespoon chopped flat-leaf parsley or rosemary

100g (3½oz) fresh baby leaf spinach
200g (7oz) potatoes, thickly sliced
2 x 150g (5½oz) fillets smoked cod, boned and skinned
1 teaspoon harissa or chilli sauce

Cook the potatoes in a saucepan of boiling salted water for 10–15 minutes, until just soft. Set aside and drain just before serving. Preheat the grill to hot. Heat the olive oil in a saucepan, add the leeks and garlic, cover and cook over a low heat for about 15 minutes, until soft but not browned. Just before serving, season the leeks and garlic with salt and pepper and add the parsley or rosemary and spinach, stirring so that the spinach wilts into the leeks. Meanwhile, smear the top of the cod with the harissa sauce. Place the cod under the grill and cook for about 7 minutes, until just firm. Place the potato slices on serving plates, spoon the leek mixture over the potatoes and serve with the cod on top.

Note: You can substitute smoked haddock for the cod. Use fresh fish if smoked is unavailable
PER SERVING: 325kcals/1370kJ 39g protein 9g fat 23g carbohydrate 8g fibre

> This makes an excellent high-protein, low-fat, low-calorie main meal with all the essential vitamins and minerals for energy production and healthy blood and immune function. The olive oil provides essential fatty acids, the spinach, leeks and potatoes vitamin C and fibre, and the potatoes the carbohydrate, making it a healthy balance for everyone. A suitable dish for wheat-, egg- and milk-free diets, you can omit the harissa or chilli sauce and use tomato purée if you suffer from digestive problems.

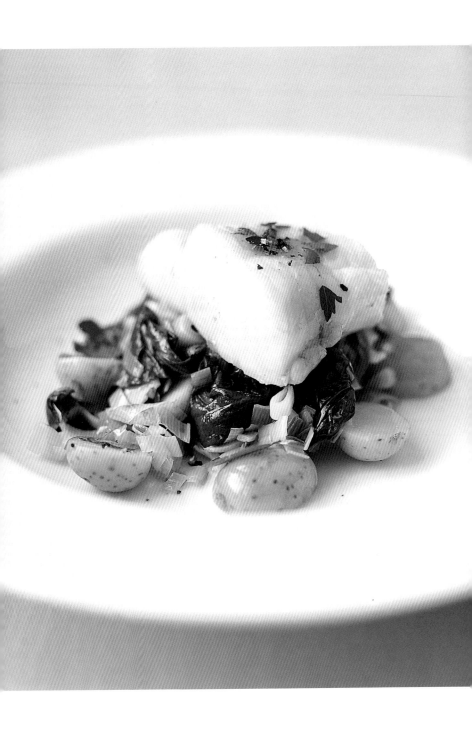

Rich in potassium, selenium, beta-carotene, vitamin E and B vitamins.

baked stuffed mushrooms

Prep time: 5 minutes, cooking time: 40 minutes, serves 2 as a light meal

2 tablespoons extra-virgin olive oil
75g (2¾oz) smoked streaky bacon,
finely sliced
1 large clove garlic, chopped
1 heaped tablespoon chopped
fresh sage

25g (1oz) wholemeal or white fresh
breadcrumbs
1 heaped tablespoon chopped fresh parsley
4 large flat field or portabello mushrooms
75g (2¾oz) goat's cheese or other firm and
creamy light cheese

Preheat the oven to 180°C (350°F/Gas 4). Heat the olive oil in a frying pan and cook the bacon over a medium heat until golden brown. Add the garlic and sage and cook for 1 minute. Add the breadcrumbs and cook for a further 1 minute until crisp. Remove from the heat and stir in the parsley.

Place the mushrooms snugly in a gratin or baking dish and divide the mixture over them. Dollop over the goat's cheese and bake for 30 minutes, until the mushrooms are soft. Serve hot or at room temperature with salad, or as part of a selection of vegetables, or on multi-grain toast rubbed with garlic and a drizzle of extra-virgin olive oil as a snack.

PER SERVING: 370kcal/1530kJ 16g protein 30g fat 8g carbohydrate 3g fibre

Serve these mushrooms with garlic bread to boost the carbohydrate content. This dish is rich in protein and energy-releasing B vitamins. It also supplies fluid-regulating potassium, immune-boosting minerals and protecting antioxidants. To reduce the fat content, use a lower fat cheese such as ricotta and dry-fry the bacon.

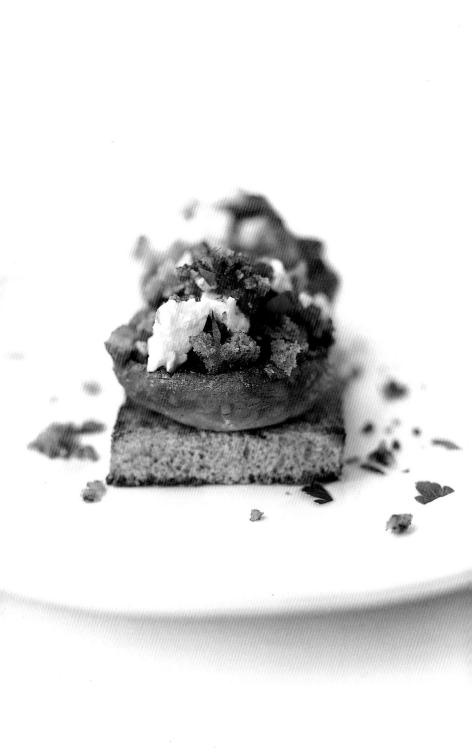

Rich in minerals and trace elements, vitamins E and C, beta-carotene and B vitamins, including folate.

cheese, walnut and spiced pear salad

Prep time: 15 minutes, cooking time: 15 minutes, serves 4 as a starter or 2 as a light meal

2 large pears
100ml (3½fl oz) balsamic vinegar
100ml (3½fl oz) red wine
Pinch of ground cinnamon
1 star anise or pinch of Chinese five spice
2 heaped teaspoons brown or unrefined brown sugar
100g (3½oz) watercress and/or spinach

3 tablespoons walnut, pumpkin seed or extra-virgin olive oil
1 tablespoon balsamic vinegar, extra (optional)
Salt and pepper, to taste
200g (7oz) soft blue cheese, such as dolcelatte or roquefort, cut into small cubes
100g (3½oz) fresh walnuts, lightly toasted
4 thin slices of toasted walnut or wholemeal bread, to serve

Peel and cut the pears into quarters, remove the cores and cut again into eighths. Place in a small saucepan and add the balsamic vinegar, wine, cinnamon, star anise or Chinese five spice, and sugar. Cover with a circle of greaseproof paper, bring to the boil and simmer gently for about 15 minutes until the pears are soft. Set aside to cool, then place in a bowl or glass jar until needed. Discard the liquid before serving.

Place the watercress and/or spinach in a bowl with the oil, balsamic vinegar if using, and salt and pepper. Mix to coat the leaves, then add the cheese, walnuts and pear slices in the bowl or serve on individual plates. Serve with the toast.

Note: A 200g (7oz) jar of spiced or pickled pears, drained, can be substituted for the cooked fresh pears if preferred.

PER SERVING (with 2 slices of wholemeal toast): 1130kcals/4690kJ 40g protein 87g fat 40g carbohydrate 9g fibre

A very high-protein, high-calorie, vitamin- and mineral-rich lunch for active people. To reduce the fat and calories significantly, use a lower fat cheese such as brie, camembert or ricotta. This recipe could be adapted for vegans by using tofu or soya cheese or for those sensitive to cow's milk by using goat's cheese. Served with rice cakes, it would also be suitable for a wheat-free diet. It is a useful dish for vegetarians as it provides essential vitamin B12 for healthy blood and energy production.

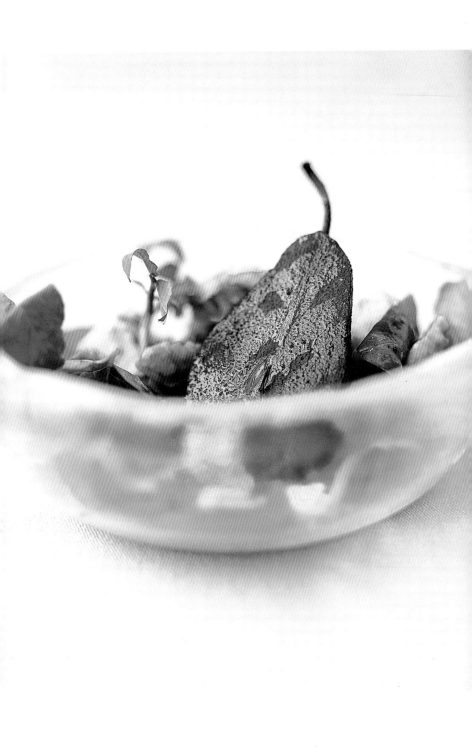

A rich source of carbohydrate, fibre, and most energy-releasing minerals and vitamins.

spinach and sweet potato crescent

Prep time: 30 minutes, cooking time: 40 minutes, serves 4

2 tablespoons olive oil
1 medium onion, quartered and thinly sliced
1 clove garlic, chopped
400g (14oz) orange-fleshed sweet potatoes, peeled and cut into 2cm (¾in) cubes
1 teaspoon grated nutmeg
Salt and pepper, to taste

300ml (½ pint) milk
1 bayleaf
250g (9oz) fresh spinach, washed
1 tablespoon cornflour (cornstarch) mixed with 1 tablespoon cold water
4 sheets ready-made shortcrust or puff pastry
Milk or beaten egg, for brushing

Heat the oil in a large saucepan and cook the onion and garlic over a medium-low heat for about 10 minutes, until soft and transparent. Add the sweet potatoes, nutmeg, salt and pepper to taste and cook for 1 minute, stirring continuously. Add the milk and bayleaf, then cover and and simmer for 10 minutes until the sweet potatoes are soft. Drain through a colander over a bowl, reserving the milk.

Briefly cook the spinach in boiling salted water, then refresh in cold water. Drain, then squeeze out as much water as possible and chop coarsely.

Pour the reserved milk back into the saucepan and add the cornflour (cornstarch) mixture. Stir continuously for 1 minute, until thickened. Combine the sweet potato mixture with the spinach and thickened milk, check for seasoning and leave to cool.

Preheat the oven to 200°C (400°F/Gas 6). Roll out the pastry thinly and cut out four circles, each 20cm (8in) in diameter. Chill for 10 minutes. Brush the outside edge of the pastry discs with the milk or beaten egg. Divide the filling and place in the middle of each pastry disc, then fold over the sides to make a crescent, pinching them together. Brush the pastry with milk or egg, place on an oven tray and bake for 15–20 minutes, until the pastry is a light golden brown. Serve hot or at room temperature, with salad.

PER SERVING: 770kcals/3200kJ 15g protein 45g fat 80g carbohydrate 11g fibre

A fibre-filled dish suitable for vegetarians. Garnish with egg or nuts to boost the protein content for a midday snack, or serve with a colourful salad of fresh green leaves and chopped yellow and red peppers (capsicums) for a carbohydrate-rich supper that will lift your mood. Homemade wholemeal pastry is a nutritious alternative to ready-made shortcrust or puff pastry.

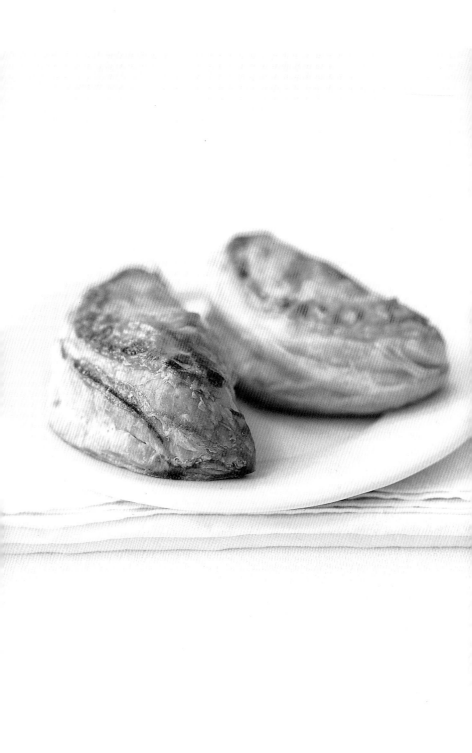

Provides a wide range of vitamins and minerals, plus essential fatty acids.

smoked mackerel salad with horseradish, watercress and green beans

Prep time: 30 minutes, cooking time: 10 minutes, serves 4

400 g (14 oz) medium-sized potatoes, cut into thick slices

150 g (5½ oz) green beans, trimmed

100 g (3½ oz) watercress or mixed salad leaves

1 fennel bulb (250 g/9 oz), halved and thinly sliced

1 tablespoon coarsely chopped fresh tarragon (optional)

Salt and pepper, to taste

1 tablespoon lemon juice or white wine vinegar

2 tablespoons extra-virgin olive oil

200 g (7 oz) peeled cooked fresh beetroot, thickly sliced then cut into strips

4 heaped teaspoons low-fat bio (natural) yoghurt

4 heaped teaspoons freshly grated horseradish or hot horseradish sauce

4 fillets (350 g/12 oz) smoked mackerel, skinned, boned and cut into large strips

Cook the potatoes in boiling salted water for about 10 minutes, until tender. Meanwhile, steam the green beans for 2 minutes, until bright green and just tender. Drain the beans and set aside to dry.

Place the watercress or salad leaves in a large salad bowl, then add the sliced fennel, potatoes, green beans and tarragon if using. Season with salt and pepper, drizzle over the lemon juice or vinegar and olive oil, and mix well.

Just before serving, add the beetroot and mix briefly, to prevent the beetroot discolouring the other vegetables.

Mix the yoghurt with the horseradish and set aside. Place the salad on individual plates and scatter over the mackerel pieces. Place a dollop of the horseradish dressing on top and serve immediately.

PER SERVING: 490 kcal/2030 kJ 22g protein 34g fat (mainly monounsaturated) 25g carbohydrate 5g fibre

Suitable for wheat-free diets, this salad is an excellent source of essential fatty acids and fat-soluble vitamins and antioxidants, providing most of the essential vitamins and minerals for energy, blood, hormone and immune functions. It is also rich in protein, making it an ideal balanced midday meal.

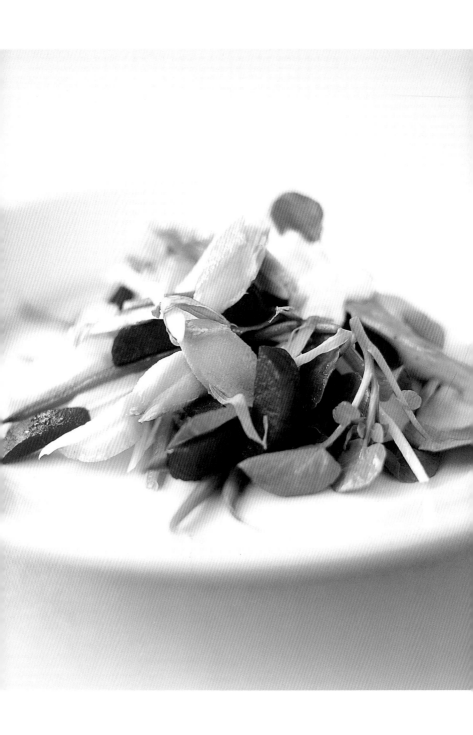

Rich in potassium, phosphorus, iron, zinc, selenium, iodine, beta-carotene, vitamins C, D, and E, and B vitamins including folate.

poached egg salad with bacon, red pepper (capsicum) and croutons

Prep time: 15 minutes, cooking time: 5 minutes, serves 4

2 large red peppers (capsicums)
150g (5½oz) mixed salad leaves, such as cos and watercress
4 spring onions, trimmed and finely sliced
1 large ripe avocado, quartered and sliced
4 medium-sized slices wholemeal bread
1 large clove garlic, peeled and cut in half
1 tablespoon sunflower oil

8 rashers smoked streaky bacon
dash of vinegar
4 eggs
Dressing:
2 teaspoons Dijon mustard
1 tablespoon white wine vinegar or lemon juice
4 tablespoons extra-virgin olive oil
Salt and pepper, to taste

Grill the peppers (capsicums) until black, and place in a sealed plastic bag to cool. Remove the skin and seeds, then cut into strips. Place the salad leaves in a large salad bowl and add the onions, avocado and peppers. Toast the bread and rub both sides with the garlic. Cut into 2cm (½in) cubes and add to the salad. Heat the oil in a frying pan and cook the bacon rashers until golden brown. Drain on kitchen towel.

To make the dressing, place the mustard and vinegar or lemon juice in a small jug or bowl and whisk to combine. Add the oil and whisk again, then set aside.

Bring a saucepan of salted water to a gentle boil. Pour in a dash of vinegar. Gently break an egg into a small bowl or cup and then pour carefully into the water. Repeat quickly with the other eggs and simmer gently for about 3 minutes for a softly poached egg. (Alternatively, cook in an egg poacher.) Remove the eggs with a slotted spoon and drain briefly on kitchen towel.

Pour the dressing over the salad, season well with salt and pepper, and toss to coat. Place the bacon and eggs on top and serve, or arrange on individual plates.

PER SERVING: 400kcal/1690kJ 16g protein 30g fat 18g carbohydrate 4g fibre

A good balance of protein, energy and nutrients makes this an ideal midday meal or substantial pre-activity snack. It contains most of the essential vitamins and minerals for energy, thyroid and immune functions. For vegetarians, omit the bacon. Use more bread to increase the carbohydrate content, and follow with a carbohydrate-rich dessert for a perfect evening meal.

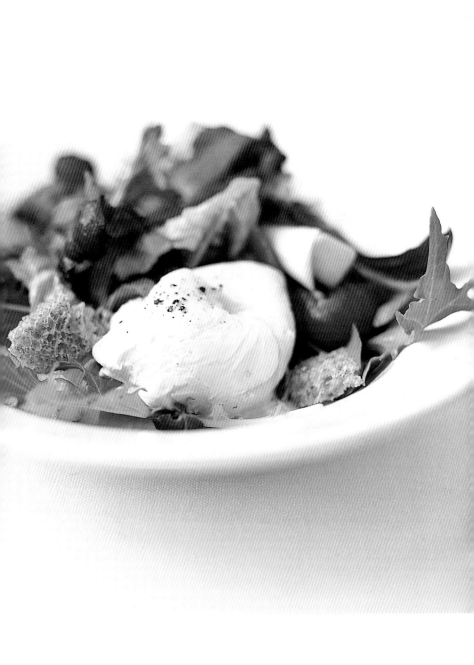

Rich in potassium, phosphorus, iron, iodine, beta-carotene, vitamins C and E, and B vitamins.

courgette (zucchini) and potato tortilla

Prep time: 10 minutes, cooking time: 45 minutes, serves 4 as a light snack

3 tablespoons extra-virgin olive oil
1 small onion, quartered and sliced
1 large clove garlic, chopped
225g (8oz) waxy potatoes, peeled and cut into small cubes
Salt and pepper, to taste

200g (7oz) courgettes (zucchini), halved lengthways and thickly sliced
4 large eggs
2 tablespoons milk
2 heaped tablespoons coarsely chopped fresh flat-leaf parsley

Heat the oil in a medium-sized frying pan, about 20cm (8in) across. Add the onion, garlic and potatoes, season with salt and pepper and cook over a low heat, stirring occasionally, for 20 minutes. Add the courgettes (zucchini) and increase the heat slightly, cooking for a further 10 minutes.

Preheat the grill to hot. Mix the eggs with the milk and add to the vegetables once the potatoes are soft. Cook for about 5 minutes until almost set, then place under the grill for a few minutes until cooked through. Set aside for 5 minutes before serving.

Serve warm or at room temperature with a salad. This tortilla makes a good substitute for a sandwich at lunchtime if you want to avoid bread.

PER SERVING: 210kcals/875kJ 9g protein 14g fat 12g carbohydrate 1g fibre

Suitable for vegetarians and wheat-free diets, this dish provides a wide range of vitamins and minerals. The potatoes provide carbohydrate and vitamin C, the courgettes (zucchini) provide fibre and the olive oil provides monounsaturated fat and vitamin E, making this a balanced snack dish. It is especially useful as a quick-to-make midday meal or light supper, followed by a carbohydrate-rich accompaniment or dessert.

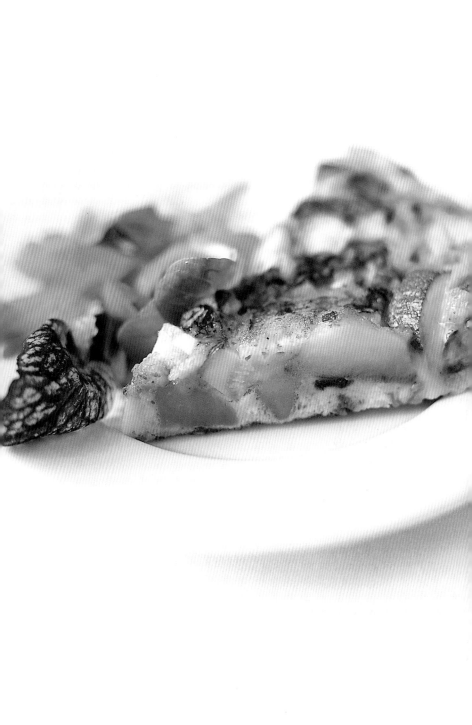

A good source of potassium, phosphorus, iron, beta-carotene, vitamins C and E, and B vitamins. Also provides essential fatty acids.

cannellini bean, red pepper (capsicum) and rocket salad

Prep time: 20 minutes, cooking time: 15 minutes, serves 2 as a main course or 4 as a starter

3 red peppers (capsicums)
1 garlic clove, crushed
zest of 1 lemon
4 tablespoons coarsely chopped fresh flat-leaf parsley

400g (14oz) cooked cannellini or flageolet beans
2 tablespoons lemon juice
4 tablespoons extra-virgin olive oil
Salt and pepper, to taste
100g (3½ oz) rocket or mixed salad leaves

Grill the peppers (capsicums) until black, and place in a sealed plastic bag to cool. Remove the skin and seeds, then cut into strips. Combine the garlic with the lemon zest and parsley. Combine the rinsed cannellini or flageolet beans with half of the parsley mixture, 1 tablespoon lemon juice, 2 tablespoons extra-virgin olive oil, and salt and pepper to taste. Place the rocket or salad leaves on a large plate and mix with the remaining lemon juice and olive oil.

Scatter the beans over the leaves, then lay the pepper strips on top, along with the remaining parsley mixture. Season with salt and pepper and serve immediately as a starter, a light meal, or to accompany grilled meat or fish.

Note: You can use a 400g (14oz) can of beans, rinsed and drained, or soak 250g (9oz) dried beans overnight then boil with a dash of oil and no salt for 30–40 minutes, until tender.

PER SERVING: 415kcals/1730kJ 14g protein 24g fat 40g carbohydrate 12g fibre

This dish is suitable for vegetarians and those on a milk-, egg- and/or wheat-free diet. Those suffering from digestive problems could serve the salad with low-fat bio (natural) yogurt. It provides slow-release carbohydrate and fibre (from the beans) to sustain energy levels, as well as B vitamins for energy production, antioxidants (vitamin C) and folate.

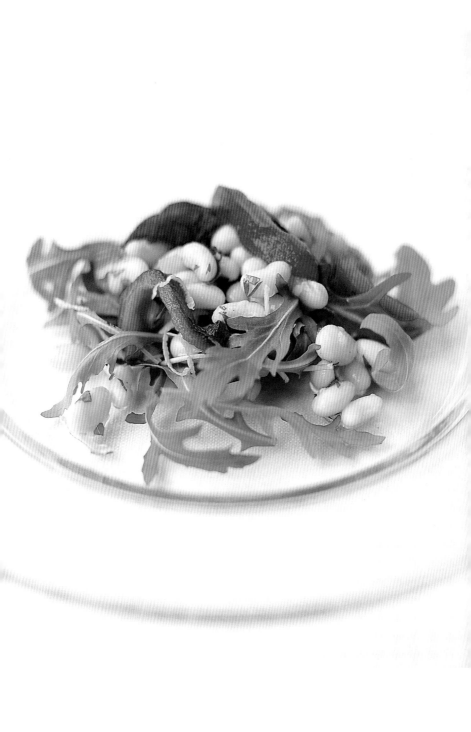

Provides potassium, vitamins A, C, D and E, folate and B vitamins.

celeriac and pumpkin dauphinoise
Prep time: 20 minutes, cooking time: 1 hour, resting time: 10 minutes, serves 4

1 heaped tablespoon chopped fresh rosemary
1 large clove garlic, finely chopped
½ large mild chilli, finely chopped,
or ½ teaspoon chilli flakes
450g (1lb) celeriac, peeled and thinly sliced

500g (1lb 2oz) pumpkin or butternut squash,
peeled and thinly sliced
Salt, to taste
570ml (1 pint) whipping cream, or half-fat
crème fraiche

Preheat the oven to 180°C (375°F/Gas 4). Mix together the rosemary, garlic and chilli. Place the celeriac and pumpkin or squash in alternating layers into a 25 x 23 x 4cm (10 x 8 x 1½ in) gratin dish, seasoning each layer with the herb mixture and some salt.

Pour the cream or crème fraiche over the top. Cover the dish with foil and bake for 45 minutes, until the vegetables are tender. Remove the foil and increase the heat to 190°C (375°F/Gas 5) for a further 15 minutes, until the dish has a nice brown crust on top. Leave to rest for 10 minutes before serving.

PER SERVING: 550kcals/2300kJ 4g protein 55g fat 8g carbohydrate 2g fibre

---

This dish is delicious on its own with just a green salad. For a complete midday meal, serve it with grilled fish, chicken or meat to boost protein and iron levels; for vegetarians, serve with stir-fried tofu or toasted nuts. To boost the carbohydrate and B vitamin content, add garlic or multi-grain bread and serve as an alternative vegetable accompaniment for an evening meal.

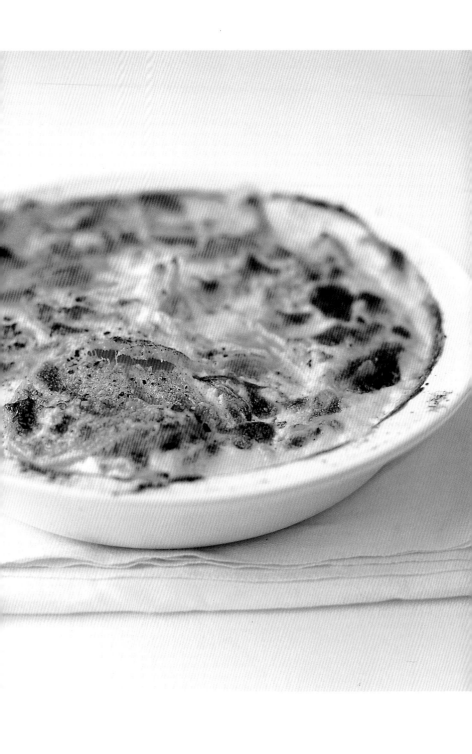

A good source of potassium, beta-carotene, vitamins C and E, and B vitamins including folate. Also high in carbohydrate and essential fatty acids.

cabbage, chestnut and ginger stir fry

Prep time: 15 minutes, cooking time: 30 minutes, serves 4

2 tablespoons sunflower oil
1 medium red onion, quartered and sliced
1 heaped tablespoon finely chopped fresh ginger
2 cloves garlic, finely chopped
325 g (11½ oz) savoy (green) cabbage, thinly sliced with any thick stems removed

200 g (7oz) chestnuts, coarsely chopped
3 tablespoons sherry or water
Salt and pepper, to taste
2 heaped tablespoons coarsely chopped fresh coriander or fresh flat-leaf parsley, to serve

Heat the oil in a wok or high-sided frying pan and cook the onion over a medium heat for 5–10 minutes or until soft. Add the ginger and garlic and cook for a few minutes more. Add the cabbage and chestnuts and stir fry for 5–10 minutes or until tender. Stir in the sherry or water and cook for a further 5 minutes. Season with salt and pepper, then sprinkle with the coriander or parsley just before serving. Delicious with plain grilled meat or fish.

Note: Boil fresh chestnuts briefly and then peel. Alternatively, ready-peeled tinned or vacuum-packed chestnuts are now widely available.

PER SERVING: 180 kcals/750kJ 3g protein 7g fat 24g carbohydrate 5g fibre

---

Suitable for vegetarians and those on a wheat-free diet, this dish is a great source of carbohydrate and essential fatty acids, antioxidants, B vitamins and vitamin C. The ginger aids digestion and the onions and garlic help the immune system. It would make an ideal snack on its own at any time of the day, or is an excellent midday meal served with meat or fish.

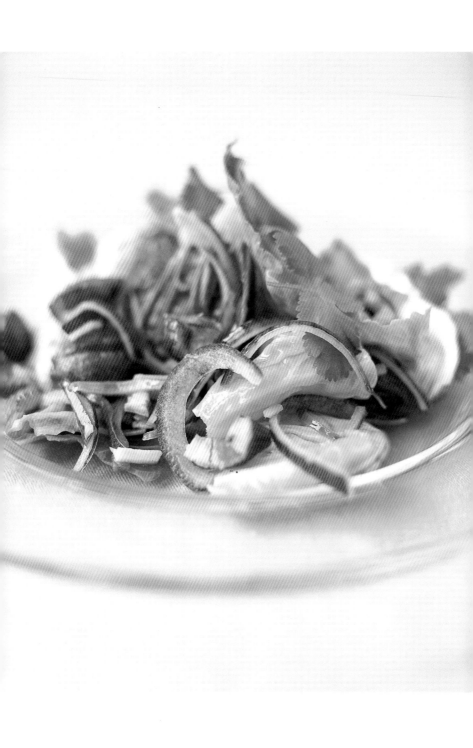

Rich in potassium, iron, beta-carotene, vitamins C and E, and B vitamins including folate, as well as essential fatty acids.

savoury potato cakes

Prep time: 10 minutes, cooking time: 30 minutes, serves 4

Olive tapenade:
100g (3½oz) good-quality black olives
2 tablespoons torn fresh basil
Zest of ½ lemon
2 tablespoons lemon juice
1 small clove garlic, crushed
Salt, to taste
50g (1¾oz) anchovies, finely chopped
½ large chilli, chopped
2 tablespoons extra-virgin olive oil
Potato cakes:
600g (1lb 5oz) potatoes

2 tablespoons extra-virgin olive oil
1 small red onion, quartered and sliced
2 red peppers (capsicums), deseeded, quartered and sliced
1 large clove garlic, chopped
1 large flat field or portabello mushroom, sliced
1 tablespoon capers, rinsed and chopped
2 heaped tablespoons chopped fresh basil
Salt and pepper, to taste
Plain flour, for dusting
Olive oil, for frying

To make the olive tapenade, remove the stones from the olives and chop coarsely. Place in a bowl and add the basil, lemon zest and juice. Mash the garlic with a pinch of salt and add with the anchovies, chilli and olive oil. Mix well and taste for seasoning.

To make the potato cakes, cut the unpeeled potatoes into quarters and boil in lightly salted water until soft. Drain and set aside. Meanwhile, heat the olive oil in a frying pan and cook the onion, peppers (capsicums) and garlic for about 20 minutes, until soft. Add the mushroom and cook for a further 5 minutes, stirring occasionally. Lightly mash the potatoes and add the onion mixture, capers and basil. Season well with salt and pepper and mix briefly. Shape the mixture into 4 large or 8 small round cakes and dust lightly with flour. Pour just enough olive oil to cover the base of a frying pan and cook over a medium-high heat for 2–3 minutes on each side, until lightly browned and heated through. Serve the cakes with the olive tapenade.

Note: Low-fat bio (natural) yoghurt mixed with coarsely chopped coriander can be substituted for the olive tapenade if you like.

PER SERVING: 440kcals/1830kJ 8g protein 22g fat 54g carbohydrate 5g fibre

These potato cakes are an excellent source of carbohydrate, as well as essential iron and antioxidants for healthy blood and body cells. They provide an ideal balance of carbohydrates for a main evening meal, or serve with yoghurt to boost protein for a midday meal or snack.

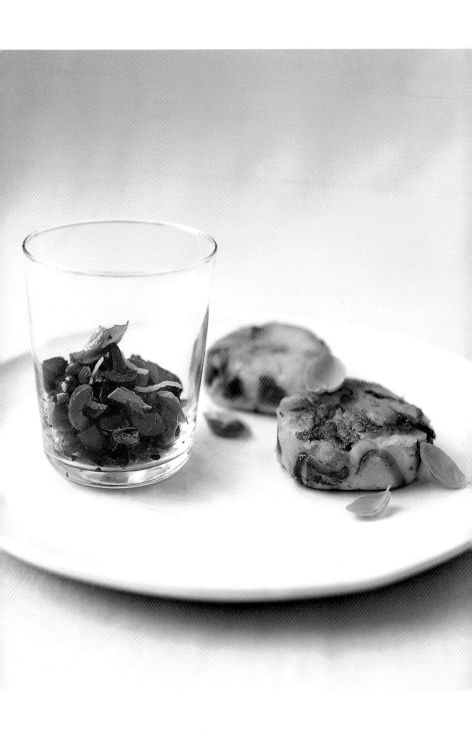

A good source of potassium, phosphorus, iron, zinc, selenium, iodine, beta-carotene, vitamins C and E, and B vitamins.

roast asparagus and potatoes with romesco sauce
Prep time: 30 minutes, cooking time: 30–40 minutes, serves 4

500g (1lb 2oz) thick asparagus
500g (1lb 2oz) small new potatoes, cut in half lengthways
4 tablespoons extra-virgin olive oil
6 unpeeled cloves garlic
Salt and pepper, to taste
Romesco sauce:
3 red peppers (capsicums)
2 cloves garlic, peeled
2 large red chillies

1 heaped teaspoon tomato concentrate (tomato paste)
25g (1oz) toasted, blanched whole or flaked almonds
25g (1oz) toasted, skinned hazelnuts
1 heaped teaspoon coriander seeds, toasted and freshly ground
4 tablespoons extra-virgin olive oil
1 tablespoon lemon juice

To make the Romesco sauce, grill the peppers (capsicums) until black and place in a sealed plastic bag to cool. Remove the skin, seeds and stem. Coarsely chop the garlic and chillies, removing the seeds from the chillies if you want a milder sauce. Place the peppers, garlic, chillies, tomato concentrate (tomato paste), nuts, coriander seeds, olive oil and lemon juice in a food processor and purée finely.

Preheat the oven to 200°C (400°F/Gas 6). Cover a roasting tray with foil. Trim the asparagus, removing the end of the stem that is tough and woody. Place the halved potatoes and asparagus on the tray, drizzle with the oil, scatter over the garlic and season with salt and pepper. Mix the ingredients together to coat the potatoes and asparagus with the oil and seasoning.

Roast the vegetables for 30–40 minutes, until the potatoes and asparagus are lightly browned and soft in the middle. Check that the vegetables are cooking evenly and turn them over half-way through cooking. Serve the vegetables with a dollop of Romesco sauce on top (any leftover sauce will keep well in the refrigerator). For a more substantial meal, serve with a poached egg or chicken breast.

Note: For thin asparagus, start cooking the potatoes and add the asparagus after 15 minutes.
PER SERVING: 440kcals/1830kJ 10g protein 30g fat (mainly monounsaturated) 31g carbohydrate 6g fibre

> These vegetables provide plenty of carbohydrate and fibre, and are very rich in vitamin C. Serve as suggested with eggs, to boost the protein levels for a balanced vegetarian meal, or with grilled lean meat to increase both iron and protein.

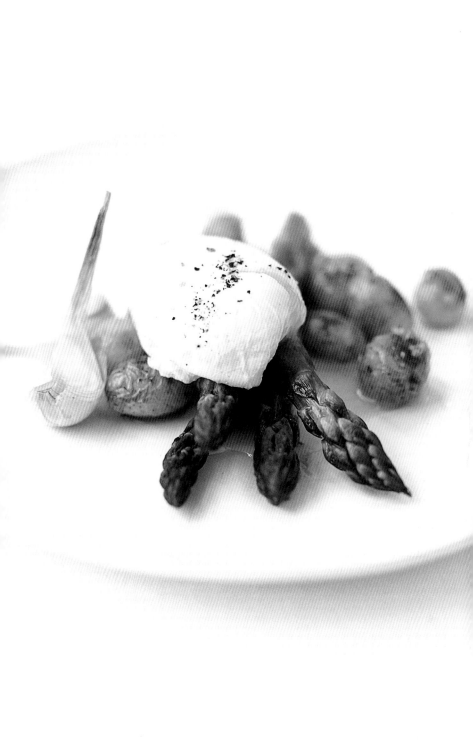

Loaded with carbohydrate and rich in calcium,
vitamin A, B vitamins and anti-oxidants.

cinnamon rice with caramelized apples

Prep time: 10 minutes, cooking time: 30 minutes, resting time: 15 minutes, serves 4

100g (3½oz) arborio or pudding rice
850ml (1½ pints) milk
75g (2¾oz) caster sugar
½ vanilla pod, split
1 small stick of cinnamon
1 strip of orange peel

25g (1oz) unsalted butter
2 eating apples, peeled, cored and cut into
16 wedges
1 heaped teaspoon brown or unrefined
brown sugar

Place the rice, milk, sugar, vanilla, cinnamon and orange peel in a heavy-based saucepan and bring to the boil. Reduce the heat and simmer gently for 20–30 minutes until completely soft and thick. Stir frequently to prevent the bottom from sticking, particularly towards the end of cooking.

Once the rice is cooked, remove the orange peel, cinnamon and vanilla and set aside to rest for 15 minutes. The rice can be cooked in advance and served either warm or chilled.

Melt the butter in a large frying pan and add the apple wedges. Sprinkle over the sugar and cook over a low heat for 5–10 minutes or until the apples are golden brown on both sides and soft. Serve over the rice.

PER SERVING: 380kcals/1580kJ 9g protein 14g fat 56g carbohydrate 1g fibre

> This dessert is ideal for boosting the carbohydrate content of an evening meal or supper dish, satisfying the biggest of appetites. It is especially useful after activity to replenish glycogen stores and carbohydrate load for active people.

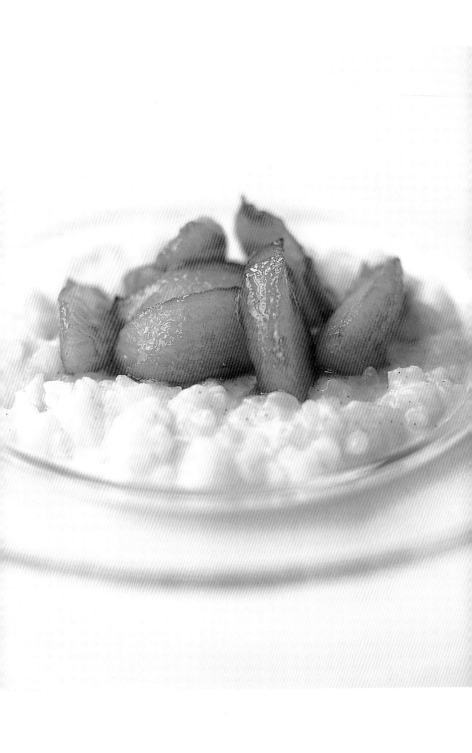

A high-carbohydrate cake rich in carotene, vitamin D, iron, and B vitamins.

carrot cake

Prep time: 20 minutes, cooking time: 40–50 minutes, serves 6

50g (1¾oz) cashew or pecan nuts, chopped and lightly toasted

3 eggs

100g (5½oz) brown sugar

250g (9oz) flavoursome carrots, peeled and finely grated

2 pieces of stem ginger, coarsely chopped

200g (7oz) Greek-style yoghurt

250g (9oz) plain flour, sieved

1 teaspoon cinnamon

1 teaspoon baking powder

1 teaspoon baking soda

150ml (5fl oz) sunflower or walnut oil

Icing sugar, for dusting

200g (7oz) low-fat bio (natural) yoghurt, to serve

Preheat the oven to 180°C (350°F/Gas 4). Grease and flour a 0.5kg (1lb) loaf tin. Whisk the eggs with the sugar until double in bulk or ribbon consistency. Peel and grate the carrots. Add the carrots, ginger and nuts to the egg mixture and mix briefly to incorporate. Fold in the yoghurt, sieved flour, cinnamon, baking powder, baking soda and oil. Pour into the loaf tin. Cook for 40–50 minutes until cooked through. To test whether the cake is cooked, push a knife or skewer into the middle of the cake and if it comes out clean it is done. Remove from the tin and cool. Dust the cake with icing sugar and serve with a dollop of yoghurt mixed with a little chopped stem ginger.

PER SERVING: 600kcals/2520kJ 12g protein 33g fat (mainly polyunsaturated) 66g carbohydrate 3g fibre

This is an ideal dessert or snack as it provides lots of carbohydrate and antioxidants to protect body cells, replenish glycogen stores. Serve with yoghurt as suggested to boost the calcium and protein content, and eat as a carbohydrate-loading snack before activity.

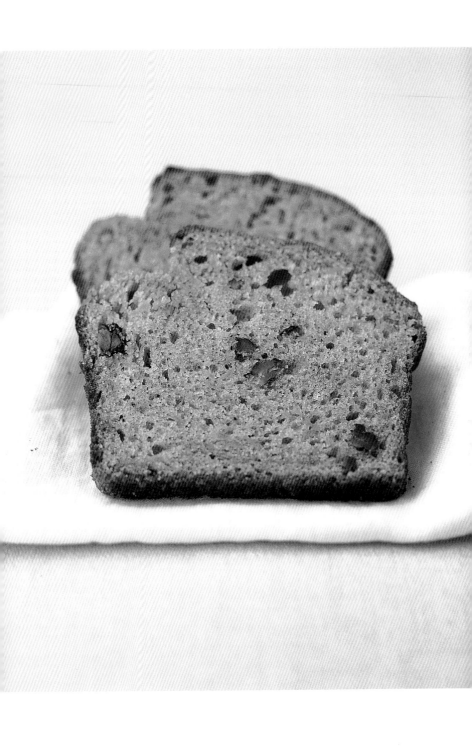

A good source of carbohydrate, with some healthy antioxidants, calcium and B vitamins.

chestnut oatcakes

Prep time: 15 minutes, cooking time: 15 minutes, makes about 12

150 g (5½ oz) softened unsalted butter or sunflower margarine
100 g (3½ oz) brown caster sugar
1 egg

100 g (3½ oz) plain flour
100 g (3½ oz) chestnuts, coarsely chopped
75 g (2¾ oz) rolled oats
Pinch of salt

Preheat the oven to 180°C (350°F/Gas 4). Line a baking tray with foil and grease lightly. Beat the butter or margarine and sugar until light and creamy, then beat in the egg.

Fold in the flour, nuts, oats and salt. Place spoonfuls the size of golf balls on the prepared tray, leaving space for spreading. Gently flatten to about 1cm (½ in) thick.

Bake for about 15 minutes, until the cakes are golden around the edges and just cooked in the middle. Transfer to a wire rack to cool. Store in an airtight container.

Note: Boil fresh chestnuts briefly and then peel. Alternatively, ready-peeled tinned or vacuum-packed chestnuts are now widely available. Substitute brazil nuts for the chestnuts if you like.

PER SERVING: 200kcal/840kJ 2g protein 11g fat 22g carbohydrate 1g fibre

These are delicious with a glass of warm milk at night to enhance sleep and replenish glycogen stores, or with a smoothie as a carbohydrate-loading snack at any time of day when energy levels are flagging.

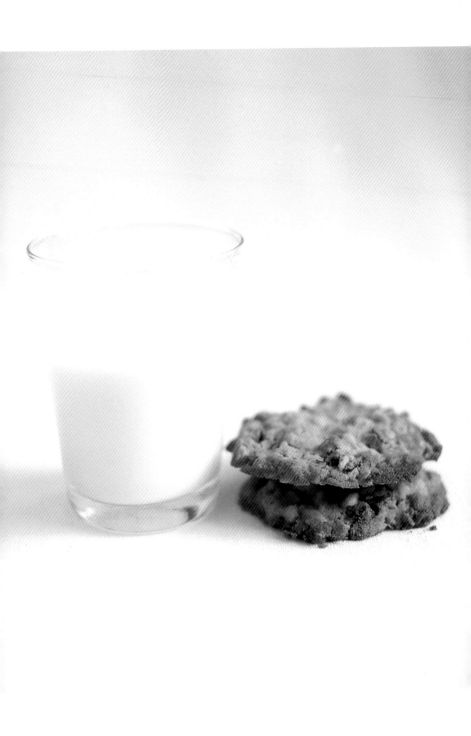

index

First published in 2002 by Murdoch Books UK Ltd. Reprinted 2003
Copyright© 2002 Murdoch Books UK Ltd

ISBN 1 903992 07 9
A catalogue record for this book is available from the British Library.

All rights reserved. No part of this publication may be reproduced,
stored in a retrieval system, or transmitted in any form or by any means,
electronic, mechanical, photocopying, recording or otherwise, without
the prior written permission of the copyright owner.

All photography by Deirdre Rooney and copyright Murdoch Books UK Ltd
except front cover top left and p7 © Adrian Weinbrecht courtesy Getty Images.

Project Editor: **Sarah Widdicombe**
Art Director: **Deirdre Rooney**
Managing Editor: **Anna Cheifetz**
Design Manager: **Sarah Rock**
Nutritional Consultant: **Susanna Holt**
Food Stylist: **Janet Smith**
Photo Librarian: **Bobbie Leah**

CEO: **Robert Oerton**
Publisher: **Catie Ziller**
Production Manager: **Lucy Byrne**

Colour separation by Colourscan, Singapore
Printed in Singapore by Tien Wah Press

Murdoch Books UK Ltd
Ferry House, 51–57 Lacy Road,
Putney, London, SW15 1PR
Tel: +44 (0)20 8355 1480
Fax: +44 (0)20 8355 1499
Murdoch Books UK Ltd is a subsidiary
of Murdoch Magazines Pty Ltd

UK Distribution
Macmillan Distribution Ltd
Houndsmills, Brunell Road,
Basingstoke, Hampshire, RG1 6XS
Tel: +44 (0)1256 302 707
Fax: +44 (0)1256 351 437
http://www.macmillan-mdl.co.uk

Murdoch Books®
GPO Box 1203, Sydney,
NSW 1045, Australia
Tel: +61 (0)2 8220 2000
Fax: +61 (0)2 8220 2020
Murdoch Books® is a trademark
of Murdoch Magazines Pty Ltd